A mother's love is a powerful force and the grief from losing a child is equally commanding. Especially when cancer preys upon child. There is no explanation why tragedies like these happen, which makes it even more difficult to accept. In this book, Shelly shares her journey with her daughter, Chantal and in doing so, puts another brick in her pathway to healing. Her book can also help other parents going through a similar experience with the threat of losing their child. Until a cure is found, we can only lean on each other for understanding and support. Thank you Shelly for opening your heart to us.

Carie Stock,
Founder and Executive Director
HELPING FAMILIES HANDLE CANCER FOUNDATION

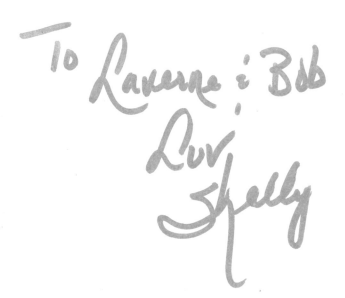

To Laverne & Bob
Luv
Shelly

I Lost my
Child to *Cancer*

A *Mother's Story*

FROM DIAGNOSIS TO HEALING AFTER LOSS

Shelly Dubois

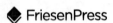

FriesenPress

Suite 300 - 990 Fort St

Victoria, BC, Canada, V8V 3K2

www.friesenpress.com

Copyright © 2016 by Shelly Dubois

First Edition — 2016

www.ILostMyChildToCancer.com

ISBN

978-1-4602-7920-5 (Hardcover)

978-1-4602-7921-2 (Paperback)

978-1-4602-7922-9 (eBook)

1. Family & Relationships, Death, Grief, Bereavement

Distributed to the trade by The Ingram Book Company

TABLE OF CONTENTS

*This book is dedicated to all
of you who have shown your utmost love and
support from the time my daughter was
diagnosed until her passing.
I am grateful for the love and support
you continue to show me until this day.
You are all kind and loving souls.*

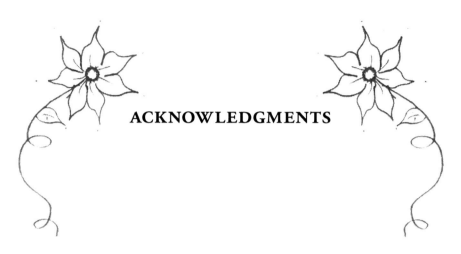

ACKNOWLEDGMENTS

Thank you to my husband of twenty-five years, Jean — your love, encouragement, and belief in me help me be who I am, and I am forever grateful that you are a part of my life.

Thank you to my daughter Aleida whose continued love and encouragement help me to be a better mother.

Thanks also to:

Friends and family who have stood by me through my worst and believe in me at my best. The universe has surrounded me with your love and support.

My hypnotherapist and friend, Barbara Adelborg. You helped save my life and for that I am forever grateful. If it weren't for you I would have never been able to continue on with living or be able to write this book.

To all those who believed in this book and in the story I have to tell. Without your financial contributions this book would not have come to print.

Chantal, you were my angel here on earth and now you are my forever angel on the other side. One day, we shall meet again.

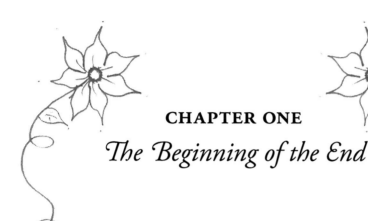

CHAPTER ONE

The Beginning of the End

IT WAS MY FORTIETH BIRTHDAY AND I was the happiest I had ever been. It was May 2006 and just ten months prior, my husband Jean and our two daughters, Chantal, then eighteen and Aleida, then fourteen, had moved from our hometown of Peace River, Alberta to Duncan, British Columbia, on beautiful Vancouver Island. I had needed a change and so had my husband. We had visited the Island a few times previously and both agreed that we wanted to live there, so we'd decided to take a leap of faith, sell our house, and move there. Aleida was not impressed to be uprooted from her friends, but Chantal was all for it even though she was in her final year of high school. We decided that she would do her first semester on the Island and then return home to Peace River to complete her final semester with all the friends she had gone to school with for most of her schooldays. We worked it out with my parents that Chantal would live with them while completing school and that after graduation, she would rejoin us on the Island.

My birthday is May fifth and Mother's Day usually falls a week or so after. On my birthday, Chantal called me and she was so happy. Graduation was just around the corner and the school year was almost over. She was healthy and loving life. Graduation was going to be "so epic"; Chantal was part of the decorating committee and she told me how they had really outdone themselves. They'd had a beautiful, grand staircase built and she was really looking forward to coming down those stairs.

That year, Mother's Day was May fourteenth, nine days after my birthday, and Chantal called again to wish me a happy Mother's Day, except this time she wasn't feeling so healthy. She said that she was experiencing blurred vision and had a really bad headache. Since I'm a migraine sufferer myself I thought maybe she had a migraine. I told her to take some Tylenol and to sleep it off.

The next morning, Chantal's headache had worsened and her blurred vision was continuing. My mother decided to take her into Emergency at the Peace River Hospital where they did a CT scan that showed a tumor in her brain. At this point, Jean and I didn't know that Mom had taken her to the hospital. Because Peace River is a small town they do not a have a MRI machine, so the doctor set up an appointment for an MRI in nearby Grande Prairie the next morning.

And then came the phone call that changed my life forever.

My mom talked to me first, and I could tell in her voice that something wasn't quite right. She explained that she had taken Chantal to the hospital, and then she handed the phone to her so Chantal could tell me the rest. Chantal requested that Jean also get on the phone. At first, Jean thought that maybe she had gotten into an accident with her vehicle. But when he got on the phone, Chantal started to cry and said, "Mom, they found a tumor in my brain."

I couldn't believe what I was hearing. I immediately started to cry, my heart sank, and panic set in. I was upset that I was unable to be there for my baby girl because she was 1400 kilometers away. Jean was just in shock and Aleida was wondering what the hell was going on. Chantal explained that she had an appointment for an MRI the next morning in Grande Prairie, and I said I would be there.

After I hung up the phone I too was in shock, and then I freaked! I had to get on a plane – I had to go. We told Aleida what was going on and she was disbelieving. Jean agreed that I had to go right away. I called my boss and explained what had just happened and she said without hesitation, "Just go. We'll take care of things."

I was on a flight early the next morning, and Jean made arrangements at work to take time off from the new job he'd started a few days before so that he and Aleida could drive out to meet us back in Alberta.

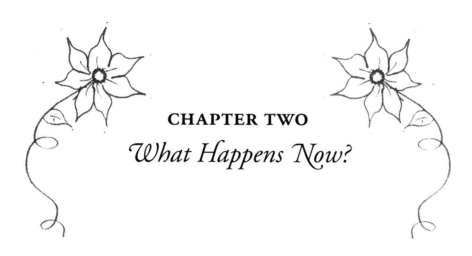

CHAPTER TWO

What Happens Now?

ALL THE WAY TO THE AIRPORT in Victoria (about an hour's drive), on the flight to Edmonton, on the layover, and then on the flight to Grande Prairie, I was in panic. I had to do a lot of self-talk to keep myself calm. Many, many things were going through my mind, and I couldn't believe that this was happening. Everything had been going so well and Chantal was so close to graduation. Things were happy and life was good! What the hell?!

During my layover in Edmonton, I couldn't stand being alone and I had to talk to somebody, so I called my long-time best friend Wendy. While I told her about Chantal I started to cry right there in the airport. I couldn't help it. I managed to keep it to a quiet cry, but I was visibly upset.

Soon it was time to get on the next plane to Grande Prairie, and I had to pull it together.

When I arrived in Grande Prairie, my sister Karen and my parents were there to greet me. The moment I saw my sister, we both burst into tears. And then I saw my parents and cried even more. Other people in the airport must have thought that I had really missed my family! Chantal was at the hospital waiting for her MRI appointment – the timing of the flight arrival and her appointment didn't quite line up. After getting my luggage we immediately went to the hospital and when I saw my baby girl I started crying, ran to her, and hugged her so tight. Being the calm kid that she was she said, "Oh Mom, get a hold of yourself. It's not that bad." Of course being a mom I couldn't stop myself from hugging and kissing her.

After Chantal's MRI, we were told that the results would be sent to a specialist at University of Alberta Hospital in Edmonton. We then returned to my parents' house in Peace River to wait for the results.

Back in Peace River, Chantal's blurred vision subsided and the headaches decreased. We hung out at my parents' place and Chantal continued to participate in preparing for graduation, which was just two weeks away.

A few days later, the doctor from the Peace River hospital called to say that she had heard from the specialist at U of A Hospital. It was definitely a tumor, located in the base of the brain – the thalamus. The specialist wanted to see Chantal right away, but because graduation was so close we made an appointment for the Monday right after it. In the meantime, Chantal was to take it easy and if she started to have a massive headache and vomiting, then she was to go to the hospital immediately.

Chantal loved to have a good time with her friends, and since it was so close to graduation there was always an activity going on. They were decorating by day and having some fun at night. I felt very protective, so I went with her to help with decorations. Then I'd let her go out with her friends for just a few hours but had her come home early to get her rest.

During this time Jean and Aleida made it to Peace River to be with us.

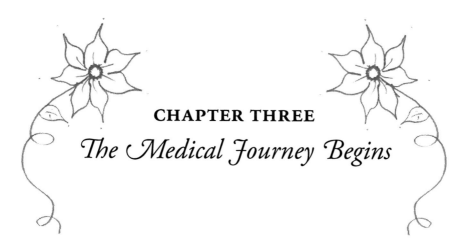

CHAPTER THREE
The Medical Journey Begins

IT WAS A WEDNESDAY MORNING AND Chantal was feeling a little lethargic and had a bit of a headache. I gave her some Advil and suggested that she sleep. And she did. And she kept sleeping. By early afternoon she was still sleeping and I was starting to be very concerned, so I went and woke her up.

We chatted for a while, she fell back asleep, and I lay there watching. Then her eyes started to flutter. I knew immediately that this was not good. We were in the basement so I ran upstairs to tell my parents that we should take her to the hospital.

When I returned to the basement Chantal was in the bathroom throwing up. I freaked! I yelled to my parents to call an ambulance.

My parents live about ten kilometers away from the hospital, and it took about twenty minutes for the ambulance to get to their house, but it seemed like forever at the time. The EMTs came down to the basement, and we managed to get Chantal to walk up the stairs and out to the ambulance. My parents and I were crying. I hugged my dad and then I got into the ambulance with Chantal.

We arrived at the Peace River hospital where the doctor on call was a friend of ours – he and my husband had played hockey together. Immediately, the nurses and the doctor started preparing Chantal to be medevac'd to U of A Hospital. I hadn't packed a bag because I hadn't been expecting to be going to Edmonton.

The team to fly her out was arriving shortly, and time was of the essence. Jean, Aleida, and my parents arrived in time to say goodbye and away in the ambulance Chantal and I went again to the local airport. There we got into a very small air ambulance plane. Holy crap. I was freaking out about Chantal and now, to add to things, I had to get into a small plane. At the time, I was not very comfortable with flying. I had done it a few times, but I was still nervous about it. So now, to get into a scary, little puddle-jumper made me very nervous, but something in me immediately overcame that fear because my daughter's life was at stake, and I had to do whatever it took. Looking back, I don't even remember that plane ride because I talked to Chantal the whole time.

We landed in Edmonton and once again were put into an ambulance and taken off to the hospital. When we arrived there I was expecting to get into the emergency room and be attended to by the specialist right away, because that's what I had been told at Peace River Hospital. I don't remember how long it took, but it was for quite some time that she lay on the gurney in the hallway, along with many others waiting to get into the Emergency Room. The EMT with us had given the papers to the admitting desk, but things were not happening very quickly.

Chantal's temperature started to rise and she started shouting about how hot she was and trying to pull her hospital gown off. I asked her to stop doing that because she would be exposing herself to everyone. She didn't care because she was so damn hot! She wanted to get up and I had to hold her and try to calm her down, and the more I tried the more upset I became. I didn't understand what was happening to her and I didn't know what to do. The EMT finally was able to get something (a drug – I can't remember what) to settle things down.

I was starting to fade because I had not eaten or drunk anything in over twelve hours, but I had to stay strong. I had to stand by my baby and help her through this.

FINALLY, the specialist came out to get her and then asked, "How long have you been out here? She was supposed to be brought in right away!"

I wanted to lose it but what good would that have done? *Let's just hurry up and get her attended to!* was my thought.

Chantal was starting to have little "freak-outs" and didn't know where she was. The specialist asked her questions like: "What is your name?" "Where were you born?" "When is your birthday?" She had to repeat herself several times before Chantal would answer.

I couldn't believe how fast this was happening. Just five hours ago we had been lying on Chantal's bed talking, and now she didn't know what day it was or where she was born!

Finally, she was taken for an MRI to assess what was happening. I sat down and I cried. I was all alone at this moment with no one to lean on. My husband and Aleida were driving out to Edmonton and had not yet arrived. It was just Chantal and me.

After the MRI they moved Chantal into Intensive Care where she was sedated and monitored. I wasn't allowed in the room until they had finished getting her all set up. When I walked in, she was hooked up to machines and lying there so still. I sat down beside her, held her hand, and talked to her. I asked her to hang on and not to give up because I loved her so much.

The nurses told me that just outside the Intensive Care Unit there was a room available for families of new patients where I could lie down. I didn't want to leave Chantal's side, but I was exhausted and had to lie down. Just for a little while. I think I managed to sleep on and off.

The next morning, a team of doctors came and spoke with me. They explained that the tumor was located in the thalamus, which is just above the brain stem. It was putting pressure on a ventricle on that area of the brain and causing a blockage of the cerebrospinal fluid, preventing it from flowing properly around the brain and spinal cord. Without a proper flow, the fluid had built up on the brain, causing the headaches and vomiting and affecting body temperature. Then they explained the procedure that they had to do to relieve the pressure of the buildup of fluid on the brain. A small hole would be drilled through the skull on the top right side of her head, and a tube inserted to drain the fluid. It was a procedure that they had performed regularly with brain tumors. They were also going to try to retrieve a piece of the tumor so that they could do a biopsy to determine whether it was benign or malignant. While they were at it, they were also going to re-route the flow of the cerebrospinal fluid. One small consolation – they said that they didn't have to shave her head – only a small area, and she could cover it up with the rest of her hair. Once the procedure was complete and she was stabilized they would come and get me to go see her.

After they left the room all I could think was, O*H! MY! GOD! They are going to drill a hole in her skull! And* I had to sit in that room and wait while they were doing this to my child. My poor kid! But I also knew that this was something that could save her life and relieve the pressure that was causing her so much grief. So I sat and waited.

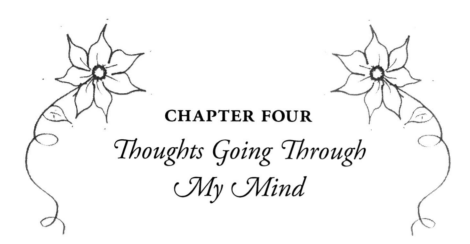

CHAPTER FOUR

Thoughts Going Through My Mind

AS I WAITED FOR THE DOCTORS to perform the procedure to relieve the pressure on Chantal's brain, I thought about many things. How much I wanted her to live was number one. But I also thought about the day she was born. My almost-New Year's baby of 1988 (one baby had been born before her) on that cold day of January second, my beautiful, little, pink bundle of six pounds twelve ounces arrived. She was so perfect. Not a flaw. Beautiful eyes, perfect lips, cute little button nose, and just a fuzz of blonde hair with a little patch of platinum-blonde on the very top of her head, which stayed that color the rest of her life. She took her time learning how to walk because she was in no hurry. She didn't walk until she was fourteen months old. She grew into a cute little blondie and was told many times by older women that she was going to break boys' hearts one day. The show *Full House* was very popular at the time and it was said to us numerous times that she looked like the little girl on the show.

I thought about all her different interests. First she'd tried playing the violin, then figure skating, piano lessons, and hip hop dance. How she loved school sports like basketball and volleyball through her junior and senior high years. But she found her true passion when she was twelve years old and her Uncle Dave took her out golfing. She absolutely loved the sport and got totally hooked. She had been in several golf tournaments and always got complimented on her beautiful swing. It was her dream to be a pro golfer one day.

I remembered all the first days of school – especially kindergarten. She was so afraid and I was so ready for her to go to school. But when it came time to actually leave her at school that very first day, I cried. So did other mothers.

A feeling of pride came through me as I recalled all her academic achievements throughout her school years as an A+ student who always worked hard at her studies. Nothing like her mother. I'd screwed around in school and did not want to be there!

There were many memories of her little group of very close friends who would continue to be her friends until her passing; Shivon, Colleen, Megan, Ashlea, Carlee, Sarah, Emma, and Michelle. They did everything together. Her friends labeled Chantal's laugh as the "trucker" laugh, and they made fun of her appetite for pyroghys and would laugh even harder when after eating them, she'd say, "Best shit ever!"

Chantal was the hair stylist for her friends for all the school dances – she sure knew how to do an up-do! She LOVED to party and always looked forward to hanging out with her girlfriends at a party. I remembered how I had loved to party as a teenager too, and I didn't have a problem with it. She was having a really good time.

She loved country music and loved to two-step! Now, she came by that honestly as I am a country singer and was playing music in bands throughout her whole life. There was nothing like going to a wedding and dancing.

Ah yes – weddings. As a little girl Chantal LOVED to play wedding. She dressed up her baby sister many times as a little bride, while she was the wedding planner – something else she aspired to do one day. She always prepared everything. I had material left over from my wedding dress, which I had hung on to (don't know why), but she would pin it all together on Aleida to make a bridal gown. Then she would do Aleida's hair, make a bouquet, and arrange my flowerpots to create an aisle for Aleida to walk down. And she had the boom box playing music. Then Chantal would be the officiant and marry Aleida to an imaginary husband. Chantal and her friend Ashlea informed me later in life that when Jean and I had band practice in our basement, they would be upstairs pretending to have a wedding dance.

All these thoughts and memories flashed through my mind in such a short period of time.

And then the doctors came to get me.

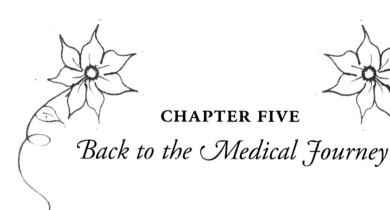
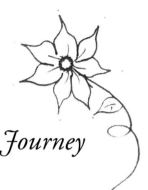

CHAPTER FIVE

Back to the Medical Journey

NO PARENT IS EVER PREPARED FOR what they are going to see when they walk into an Intensive Care Unit and see their child lying there. Chantal had a tube coming out of her head, arterial lines hooked up to her arm, and monitors for her heart and body temperature.

A lot of the pressure on Chantal's brain had been relieved because of the fluid having been drained. While accomplishing this, her team of doctors had also managed to somehow reach the tumor to get a piece of it for biopsy, and they had rerouted the cerebrospinal fluid around the tumor. The tumor was officially considered inoperable because of its location in the brain – in the thalamus. Now all I could do was sit by her side and wait.

When Chantal finally awoke, the nurse was right there to start asking questions: "What is your name?"

She knew that.

"What day is it?"

She didn't know.

"What year is it?"

I think she said, "Nineteen something."

"Where were you born?"

She said, "Peace River."

"Who is your mom?"

She turned her head, pointed to me, smiled and said, "She is."

That made me smile so big, and I cried joyful tears.

It was a Thursday and graduation was in two days. Since Chantal didn't know what day or year it was, I wasn't going to tell her that she would miss graduation. It didn't seem important just then anyway.

Every day there was progress. Chantal became more alert and aware of her surroundings and of what was going on. Family and friends were visiting on a continual basis, and she was happy to see everyone. It didn't take long before she was sick of hospital food, so a Subway sandwich and a few other things made their way to her. She was pretty happy about the Subway sandwich.

Jean and Aleida made it over from Peace River, and my parents and sister Karen also arrived, along with Chantal's boyfriend, Matthew.

Chantal finally improved enough that we started staying at a nearby hotel for the evenings, returning early each morning. We stayed at the hospital day in/day out, playing cards, doing puzzles, and just hanging out. When Chantal finally started knowing what day and year it was, she soon realized that she had missed her graduation, which upset her greatly. Like any student who had finally completed twelve years of schooling, she had been really looking forward to this day, and she had missed it. Some of her best friends, Shivon, Emma, and Michelle came to visit her, and they brought gifts and pictures to show her. Everyone had signed a picture and there were lots of get-well notes.

The day arrived that Chantal was well enough to leave the Intensive Care Unit and move to another room. We were all so pleased and grateful.

Ten days went by and Chantal was released, but before she left the specialist saw her. He explained that the biopsy tests of the tumor had not been completed and that he wanted us to stay in the city for another week to be on the safe side. Relatives in nearby St. Albert graciously opened their home for us to stay. After a couple more days, Jean and Aleida had to return back to the Island – Jean had to go to work and Aleida went back to school.

After a week we had another appointment with the specialist, and because the results were *still* not back he did not want us returning to

British Columbia. He said we could go back to Peace River and wait there for his phone call.

Back in Peace River we stayed at my parents' house once again and patiently waited for the phone call from the doctor. Finally, after almost a week had gone by, the call came. My mom answered the phone and the doctor asked to speak to Chantal. As she spoke with him, my parents and I watched her face light up and she looked like she was getting happier by the second. When she hung up the phone, she said with such excitement, "The tumor is NOT cancerous!"

We all shouted for joy and we were so relieved!! Everything was going to be fine!

After all the excitement settled down, I asked her what else the doctor had had to say. He'd explained to her that sometimes people can get tumors and they are not always cancerous. Because hers was benign and inoperable, it was just something she would have to live with.

We were satisfied.

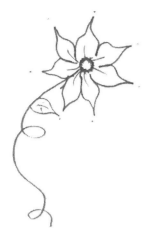
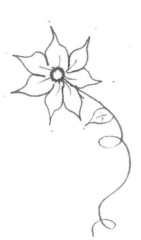

CHAPTER SIX

Graduation

SINCE CHANTAL HAD MISSED HER BIG graduation day, I thought it would be a good idea to have a graduation party. It was a great way to celebrate that she was alive and that she could have a celebration with her friends and family.

I booked the local Legion Hall in Peace River and I invited all our relatives who lived in the area and all of her closest friends. We did a potluck and I even ordered a cake with her graduation picture on it. There were many comments about how much Chantal looked like me in her graduation picture, which was very flattering. I had also made arrangements with the principal and vice principal of her school to bring a graduation gown for Chantal and to present her with her high school diploma. They wore their academic regalia as well! Even though it wasn't her "actual" graduation day, since she was presented with her diploma and all of her girlfriends got dressed up again in their graduation dresses, it was a perfect day. One of the teachers had supplied some of his old cars for the original graduation day, and he very thoughtfully brought a car to Chantal's party too. Lots of pictures were taken in and around the car. It was a beautiful event and I was so grateful that it all came together.

A few days later, we returned to our home in BC.

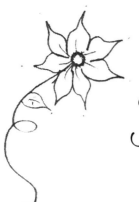
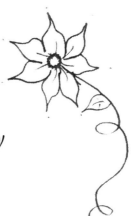

CHAPTER SEVEN

Another Biopsy
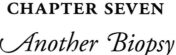

WE WEREN'T HOME A WEEK BEFORE I looked at Chantal and said, "There is something wrong with your eyes. Something is not right." She said that she really didn't think that anything was wrong so I left it alone. A few days later, her vision started becoming blurry again. Oh God! We had thought everything was fine. What the hell was happening?

I took her into Emergency right away at Cowichan District Hospital, which was only five minutes from where we lived in Duncan. Once I explained what had previously happened to Chantal, they immediately sent us to Victoria General Hospital to see a specialist. Here we go again.

Chantal was admitted right away and was given a bed, but we waited four days until the specialist came to see her. The specialist was so busy he didn't have time to take Chantal on as a patient, so he finally referred her to another specialist who was able to come and see her. I was frustrated with having to wait around, but we were told by the nurses that if we left we would lose the bed and would have to wait even longer to see a doctor.

This specialist consulted with the specialist at U of A Hospital and he then explained to us that he was going to perform another biopsy.

He said that he had to go through the side of her head in front of her right ear to get a larger piece of the tumor. Another surgery. Another sit...and wait...

When they brought Chantal back from surgery, she had a huge bandage on the side of her head. They'd had to shave off quite a bit of her long, beautiful hair in that area but it was something that had to be done.

A few days later, the specialist dropped by to see her and informed us that Chantal could go home. He explained that whether the tumor was benign or cancerous we would receive a phone call from BC Cancer Agency with the results. Once again, we waited for a phone call.

A few days after her release it was Canada Day and Chantal wanted to go to the celebrations at the harbor and parliament building in Victoria. She didn't care that she had a huge Band-Aid on the side of her head. To put it bluntly, she really didn't give a shit. She just called it her "war wound." She wanted to have fun and no one was going to stop her.

I can't remember how long we waited for that phone call, but it finally came. We had an appointment at BC Cancer Agency for the results.

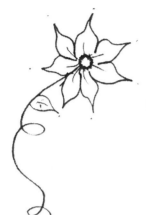
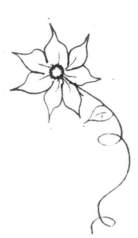

CHAPTER EIGHT

It's Cancer

AS WE PARKED THE CAR AND entered the building at BC Cancer Agency, Chantal and I were both quite nonchalant about the whole ordeal. Today we were going to find out the results of the biopsy... but we were not prepared for what we were about to hear.

A doctor with a very thick French accent, began by giving us treatment options. I said, "Treatment options? Why?"

He then asked us, "Were you not told the results of the biopsy?"

I said, "No. That's why we are here."

He sighed with some disbelief and then proceeded to inform us that the tumor was indeed cancerous and that it was a Glioblastoma Multiforme, also known as Stage IV Astrocytoma – the worst kind. The doctor went on to explain that this type of tumor was the most common and the most aggressive, and therefore they wanted to start treatment immediately.

Chantal and I looked at each other with shock, disbelief, and fear in our eyes. How could this be? What next? Were we going to be told that she didn't have long to live?

Oh my God!! What is happening?? They'd just told us at U of A Hospital that it was benign and now we were being told it was cancerous at Stage IV – and this was only three weeks later! I was not only in shock and disbelief, I was now mad!! How the fuck could they miss this before?

As the doctor continued to explain the treatment protocol, Chantal and I just cried and didn't absorb anything he was telling us. *All of a sudden she has to start chemotherapy and then radiation* – our heads were spinning. The chemotherapy treatment was to be administered by pill form so we had to go to the pharmacy in the Cancer Institute and get the pills. The pharmacist said it would be about an hour, so Chantal and I walked outside.

We were speechless and kind of walked around aimlessly. What the hell had just happened in there? If I had known we were going to be told it was cancer I would have had Jean come with us as well. But we'd thought it was just an appointment! Cancer? Stage IV? What was going to happen to my poor baby? I don't know what was going through Chantal's mind, because she really didn't say anything. I think she was in total shock as well.

Overwhelming is the word. Chantal had just been diagnosed with Stage IV brain cancer, information was being flung at us, we were getting pills to start chemo, and in a few weeks she would have to start radiation for a full six weeks.

We drove from Victoria back to Duncan (about a forty-five minute drive), and I can't even remember the drive home. I can't remember if Jean was home from work or Aleida was home from school, but I do remember telling them and we all just sat and cried. I tried to explain to Jean all that had happened at the Cancer Agency, but everything was still in such a blur. I don't retain information at the best of times, and this time was definitely no exception. We then called family and friends to inform them of the news.

We had another appointment at the Cancer Agency, where we would meet with a counselor to help prepare us for what Chantal would be going through. We would also meet with the oncologist and radiation therapy specialist. The oncologist was a nice, soft-spoken man, and he was very tender with his words towards Chantal. He knew how devastated she was and so he tried very hard to keep the conversation "light," explaining about the chemotherapy drugs and another drug– Dexamethasone. He also broke the news to her that because of the chemotherapy, her hair was going to start falling out and he suggested cutting it short. For a girl who'd had long hair all her life, that was just another blow.

We then saw the radiation therapy specialist and he explained the treatment protocol for radiation. There would be six weeks of daily radiation treatments (except for weekends).

We now had a list of appointments, drugs that had to be administered, and a radiation treatment plan. But this was all in Victoria and we lived in Duncan. Both my husband and I were working full-time jobs, and I had already missed a lot of work just a month before while Chantal was in the Edmonton hospital. How were we going to manage this?

The morning after we'd been given the diagnosis, I returned to work. My boss at the time asked how things had gone. I teared up and told him that it was cancer and that I didn't know what to do because of all the upcoming appointments, etc. We worked it out that I could work part time – that I would work mornings and then have the afternoons off. My income was now cut in half.

Since I had been a hairdresser back in the day, Chantal asked me to cut her hair. I did not want to be the one to do it, but she insisted. She pulled out my scissors and my cape and said, "Let's do this."

I tried so hard to be upbeat about the whole ordeal, but with each snip I felt a pang in my heart. Yeah, I know it's only hair and it will grow back. But it wasn't going to grow back! I was cutting her hair because it was going to start falling out! Not a great feeling. I held back the tears as the locks of beautiful, blonde hair fell to the floor. Both Aleida and I had long hair at the time, so to be supportive we cut our hair off as well.

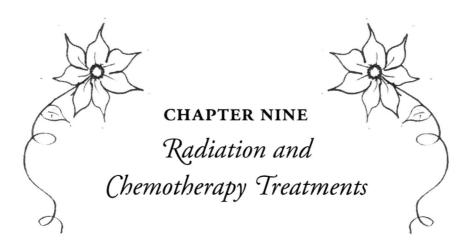

CHAPTER NINE

Radiation and Chemotherapy Treatments

AT THIS POINT, CHANTAL WAS ONLY taking the chemotherapy drugs, and she was enduring them well without major sickness. It was time for radiation treatments. The first appointment was to have "the mask" made. When an individual receives radiation treatments to the head area, a mask is custom-made to your face. It is used to make sure your head remains perfectly still while a precision beam of high-energy radiation is targeting the tumor. Many radiotherapy departments use a type of plastic mesh called thermoplastic to make the masks. This mesh is soft when warm and hardens as it cools. The warmed plastic is shaped to your face and head. It does not cover your nose or mouth, so you can breathe easily. When the plastic cools it creates an exact impression of your face and head.

Doctors quite often use radiotherapy to treat brain tumors. Because the radiation treatments caused swelling, Chantal had been prescribed Dexamethasone – a drug that I came to hate. Dexamethasone helps reduce swelling around the affected area. Weird thing though – it might help with inflammation, but because it increases your appetite immensely, you can't stop eating and it's constant. Another side effect – it makes your body balloon up. Within no time, Chantal's perfect, little, thin body became larger and larger – her face getting puffier and puffier. Stretch marks developed on her inner thighs, her waist, under her arms, and around her breasts. I had never seen so many stretch marks – not even on a pregnant woman. Because the weight gain happened incredibly quickly, the stretch marks were so deep that they actually started to bleed. I had to bandage them and try to comfort her in her discomfort. Not only was she getting the stretch marks, though, her hair had started to fall out. With every hair wash, clumps of hair fell out and then combing was no different. My heart sank with every handful, but Chantal held her head high and persevered. As each week of radiation treatments passed by, she also started to become wobbly because her balance was affected. We had to help her up the stairs and assist with other minor functions. How I hated to watch this happening to her. Even though she was showing strength on the outside, I knew how she hated it as well.

It was now July, it was extremely hot that summer, and the further we got into the treatments, the more tired she became. The heat was becoming unbearable for her. Not only was it hot, but then road construction started on the street right in front of our house and continued for weeks. Because it was so hot we had to leave the windows open and endure the noise while Chantal was trying to sleep. At least the more tired she got, the easier it was to fall asleep, and eventually it didn't matter how hot or noisy it was.

I can't remember how I came to learn of a product called Oncolyn, which was created by a Dr. Arthur Djang. Oncolyn slows down free radicals' injury to normal tissue and enhances cellular immune function for the destruction of cancer cells. It also possesses the capacity to induce differentiation of cancer cells back toward normal cells. And it could be used in conjunction with chemotherapy drugs. I thought, *Great! This sounds like a great product! I* talked with the oncologist about it and although he wasn't aware of its ingredients he felt it could be something to try. So I ordered some and beginning in September 2006, Chantal started taking Oncolyn.

Because I was working mornings, I had to leave Chantal on her own but this became tougher and tougher to do because she was starting to not remember things. As well, her appetite had increased substantially due to the Dexamethasone, so I could no longer leave her alone.

The stress for me at having to leave her by herself was unbearable. Fortunately, some of her friends (at different intervals) decided to come visit, which helped out a great deal. Ashlea came out for about a week and then Sarah for a few days. Jean tried to take time off as well, but he had just started his new job, didn't get any vacation time because he was working a casual position, and had already missed two to three weeks when Chantal had been in the hospital in Edmonton. It wasn't that we didn't want to take time off, we couldn't afford to. We still had to put food on the table and gas was getting expensive from driving back and forth to Victoria. I had no choice but to once again take a leave of absence from my job, and we were down to one income. At this point, we still had money from the sale of our house in Peace River, but we really didn't want to touch it because it was for a down payment on the next house and we were currently renting.

Six weeks of radiation treatments were finally over. Chantal had become very lethargic and was sleeping much of the time. She had lost a lot of hair, gained a whopping fifty pounds, and her motor skills and balance had been affected. We had some family and friends come to visit, but visiting with Chantal was in intervals as she was too tired.

Now that the radiation treatments were complete it was time for an MRI to see what was happening with the tumor. Results – It had started to shrink and we were elated!! The oncologist was very happy with the results as well. Radiation therapy can only be administered for six weeks, but the chemotherapy continued.

It was now October and Chantal was recovering from the radiation treatments. She was starting to walk up stairs again without assistance, and she was able to stop taking the Dexamethasone. Her appetite was returning to normal and the weight began to come off.

We were feeling very good about things at this point. Since the tumor had shrunk and Chantal was feeling better, we felt we were gaining and were winning the war on this cancerous brain tumor. So, we had a little fun with the radiation mask. Because it was no longer needed, we wanted to destroy it, so we had her run it over with the vehicle – several times. It was pretty funny to watch her back up over it, drive forward over it, and so on. Afterwards, our dog Presley got hold of it and was running around with it in his mouth and shaking it around. We videotaped the entire thing and then Jean put music to it with the song "Eye of the Tiger."

CHAPTER TEN
Life Returning to Some Normal

I RETURNED TO WORK FULL-TIME AND since we were renting, we started looking for a new home. One day, Jean was helping out Aleida's class with a bottle drive. He drove into a new subdivision and there he saw what he felt was our new house. When he and Aleida came back home they were both so excited. Jean told Chantal and me that he felt that he had found our new home and that he wanted to take us there right away so we could see it. It was still under construction but we had a look around and really liked it. It was backed onto a green space that had walking trails and a creek below. It would be perfect! We contacted the builder and made an offer on it right away. On December 15th, 2006 we moved into our new home.

By January 2007, Chantal was feeling much better and was actually starting to feel bored. Since she couldn't work she wanted to do something. The plan before all this had happened was for her to go to the University of Victoria, work on a Bachelor of Commerce degree, and hopefully get on the university's golf team. Because she couldn't attend full-time yet, she decided that she would take some courses by correspondence to help prepare her for university. While she was taking these courses, she wrote a short story about hoping to find a cure for cancer. It was entitled "Everyone Deserves a Lifetime," and she entered it into a writing contest for which submissions came from all over North America. Her story was chosen as one of the top five percent and was published in a book called V*oice of the Future*. We were determined that she was going to win this cancer battle, therefore we kept moving forward with our lives.

Chantal was now on a break from chemotherapy so over the next few months, she continued to work on her correspondence courses, went out with friends, and was starting to live a normal life again. Regular checkups and MRIs were showing that the tumor was still shrinking.

She was also very appreciative of how much I had been there for her. That didn't matter to me. I was doing what any mother would do when her child was sick. I didn't need any thanking, but she wrote me the most beautiful letter on Mother's Day and to show you her character I have to share it with you. If only you could see it in her handwriting, for she had beautiful handwriting like mine. The flower on the cover of this book is the flower she drew on the envelope the letter was in, and she also drew a few smaller ones on the letter.

"To my Mom on Mother's Day!

There are no words to express my gratitude for you the past 19 years. You've helped me overcome, conquer and celebrate so much that has gone on through the years. People always say you're just like your Mom. I used to hate hearing it, but I knew that it was the truth and as I get older, I appreciate how lucky I am that it is you that I take after. We've had a few bumps along the way, haven't we? But I know we're going to overcome, conquer and celebrate whatever comes our way, and we know there will be more to come – that's life! Whatever I have done to make you angry, I'm sorry and please forgive me. Whatever I have done to make you sad, please forgive me for it was not on purpose. But whatever I have done to make you so full with joy and happiness, please don't ever let me stop. You're a mother who deserves the very best. So on this Mother's Day, I wanna thank you from the bottom of my heart for you! I wanna thank God and Grandma and Grandpa for you!

Because you are the best thing in my life. I love you so much and I am so thankful that I have a mother who loves me so much too. For a beautiful mother have a beautiful Mother's Day!

Love Always and Forever,
Chantal xoxo

And if I ever become a Mom, I hope I am half of what you have been to me! I love you!

I read this letter every Mother's Day.

Chantal was missing her friends back in Peace River and really wanted to go and see them. This involved flying, which I was not very comfortable with. We checked with the oncologist who said that there would be no harm in it, so we made the decision that she would go home for a few weeks. Even though the doctor said it was okay, I still wasn't okay. I had become very protective and wanted to be around her almost all the time. Even though the tumor had shrunk the way it had, I was still scared for her health and her safety.

It was really hard to put her on that plane and see her go away from me. Fourteen hundred kilometers away from me – where I couldn't watch her to make sure she ate right and took proper care of her health. Good thing there wasn't texting at that time – I would have been texting her every five minutes!

She really enjoyed her trip home to see her friends and family. It was something she needed to do even though I had a hard time with it. So I was very, very happy when she returned home.

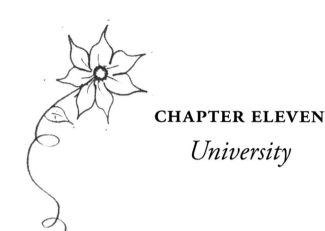
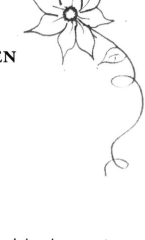

CHAPTER ELEVEN

University

IN THE SPRING OF 2007, CHANTAL was determined that she was going to university to take her Bachelor of Commerce. I was very apprehensive about her going. She still had that tumor in her brain, and even though it was small it was still there. I pleaded with her that I didn't want her to go, that I wanted her to stay home until the tumor was completely gone. I knew she was bored and needed to do something, but I didn't want her to have any stress of any kind. She finally convinced me that she should at least apply to see if she got accepted.

In June, that damn letter of acceptance came in the mail. She was so happy and I have to admit I was happy for her too, but at the same time I was still very unsure. We talked to the oncologist at a checkup and told him of her intention of going to university. He encouraged it, but he also stated that he wanted her to take a lighter course load to keep her stress level down. We met with a counselor at the university and told her of Chantal's situation. She managed to get a lighter course load for Chantal, but of course told her that it would take longer to get her degree. That, we didn't have a problem with. Usually, first-year university students have to live in the dorm, but since we proved that Chantal had a medical situation, she was able to get into an apartment on campus that she shared with three other girls.

After I had been off work for some time, funds weren't as good and in order to help pay for university, Chantal applied for a scholarship through the Servus Credit Union, which was available for students who were going into a Bachelor of Commerce program. She wrote quite the letter! There were only ten recipients to get a $2500 scholarship towards their studies and she succeeded in being one of them. The Servus Credit Union even had a special banquet to award the recipients. I was so very proud of her. And she was proud of herself. And because she had been such a good student in high school, she also received academic scholarships towards university.

That summer, we prepared for Chantal going to her first year of university. We purchased kitchen items, school supplies, and all the other things to get her set up for living on campus. Then the day came to take her to university. I tried to stay very upbeat about the whole thing – being excited that she was going to school and was going to experience university life. To a certain extent I was happy that she was going to experience this new adventure, but at the same time, there was still that friggin' tumor in her brain. I still felt the need to take care of her until she was cured. And I did not want to let that go.

As we were moving everything in we also met her new roommates. The girls picked their rooms and decided where to put things in the cupboards and in the fridges. We got Chantal's room set up and then it was time to leave. I cried. I could not help myself. But because Chantal was so strong and so determined, a small piece of me knew that she could take of herself. Thank goodness we only lived forty-five minutes away. That gave me some comfort as well.

By the second night she called, crying. Chantal has always been one to love going away, but at the same time can be very homesick. Especially now – when we had grown even closer together. It was so damn hard to hear her crying on the phone. If she hadn't still had the tumor it would have been different. But as hard as it was, and trying not to cry myself, I had to talk her through this. Oh, how much I just wanted to get into the car and go get her, but as much as I hated it I had to do some tough love. I reminded her of how insistent she had been that she wanted to do this and that it was only the second day. Even though she had three roommates, she didn't know them yet and she was by herself in her room. Being alone was something she had always disliked since she was a child. I promised her that I would come and visit on the weekend and that we would go and do something together.

As the weeks went by and Chantal started to get to know her roommates and other people, she settled in more. Her course load was manageable and she was living a normal life. In one of her courses, there was a "personal change project" and Chantal participated. She had to write an essay as to why she was going to exercise and eat healthy, and then she had to track her progress. Of course she had to customize her level of activity due to her health. One thing she said in her essay is quite profound for a nineteen-year-old going through cancer: "What I have learned is that life will throw storms along your way, but it's what you do when that storm comes that makes all the difference."

I made sure that I visited her every weekend or we would bring her home for the weekend, depending on what she had going on. A few times, when we weren't able to go get her, she even took a Greyhound bus home to Duncan.

It was so nice when Christmas holidays finally rolled around and she was home for two weeks. Because we were living fourteen hundred kilometers from our families, we had missed a couple years of going home for Christmas. That year we had saved enough air-miles and had booked our flights earlier in the year so we could go home.

We had a wonderful visit with our families. It was great for Chantal to hang out with her cousins again and to play their favorite card games of "Asshole and Spoons." The kids played games they had been playing since their early teens.

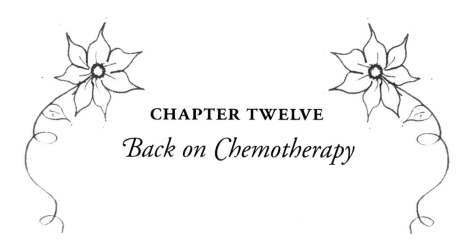

CHAPTER TWELVE
Back on Chemotherapy

IT WAS NOW JANUARY 2008, AND we had a checkup appointment with the oncologist. He was happy that Chantal was feeling fine and finding that her university course-load was manageable for her. As part of the checkup he also ordered another MRI. One thing with the medical system, when you have a brain tumor, you don't wait very long for an MRI – they are done pretty much the next day.

A few days after the MRI, the oncologist wanted to see us again.

Not good news. The original tumor had started to grow again and now…there was a second one.

Everything had been progressing so well!! Why? Why did it start growing again? And another one? What the hell!!! After all those happy moments of the tumor shrinking and Chantal feeling so well, we got *this* news. This meant that she had to go back on chemo. I really wanted to pull her out of school and bring her home, but she insisted that she wanted to continue and finish the semester. The oncologist put her back on pill-form chemotherapy (Temedol) and strongly urged her to take it easy.

And so she continued with her studies and continued to take chemotherapy. Even though not feeling very well some days, she still attended classes and managed to get her assignments completed. Now that's determination. Nothing was going to stand in her way – not even a brain tumor and chemotherapy.

February came and it was reading week, and of course I brought her home to rest. But she didn't want to rest too much. That was boring! So two of her favorite cousins, Megan and Amanda (who are sisters) came out to visit. Jean's sister Sylvia and her husband Hervey also came out to visit. We had a house-full but we were happy to see some family. We toured the Island a bit and Chantal, Megan, and Amanda were their crazy usual selves. They had a great time.

Reading week was over, Chantal went back to school, and before you know it April had arrived and then school was out. I was so happy to bring her home. Chantal was still on chemotherapy but doing well.

Chantal wanted to get on the university's golf team in her second year. So she decided that since she was finished school she would go golfing at one of the local golf clubs. It was there that she met a golf pro and after some conversation, he took her under his wing and began coaching her and giving her free golf lessons.

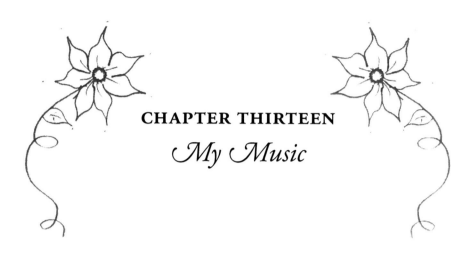

CHAPTER THIRTEEN
My Music

BEFORE CHANTAL BECAME ILL, I HAD planned on forwarding my music career and recording a CD. I had big hopes and dreams of making it famous in the country music industry. Shortly after we had moved to Vancouver Island, I began attending local jam sessions so I could meet other musicians, and I started writing songs to record. I was in my element as I had started to know many musicians, and it wasn't long before I was invited to join a band that had a traditional sound that I loved. I was playing music every Friday night, and I was having so much fun. Everything was going in the right direction. But of course everything had been put on hold when Chantal was diagnosed. When she went to school, she'd strongly urged me to continue with my music again and to record my CD. At first I didn't want to, not only because I still wanted to make time for her even though she was feeling better and going to university, but because I felt we couldn't afford it. Jean and I had both missed so much work already, but we were both back to work full-time and living somewhat comfortably again. Chantal really wanted me to do something for m*e* and kept encouraging me, and so finally I did. I had started recording in October 2007, but in January 2008 when Chantal's follow up MRI showed another tumor, I was going to put everything on hold. She strongly encouraged me to keep going. She was bound and determined to finish her semester and she wanted me to complete my CD too. By May 2008, my CD was complete and ready for release.

I had my CD release party on May 31, 2008 and Chantal was there to celebrate. I was so happy that she had encouraged me to get back to music.

CHAPTER FOURTEEN
The Start of the Decline in Health

DURING THE MONTH OF MAY, CHANTAL continued to golf and to get golf lessons from the pro. After coming back from a lesson she was always very excited about how much she was improving. She felt so good that along with some close friends we even participated in the local Relay for Life on June fourteenth and fifteenth. The weekend after, when my parents came to visit, Chantal went to the driving range with Jean and my dad and noticed that her swing wasn't as good. A few days later, she went out golfing with the pro again and when she came back she commented that her swing wasn't very good – that it was really weak. A few days later, her left side really started to weaken, so I called the oncologist and made an appointment. He ordered another MRI for her to have done before seeing him.

Chantal started becoming very tired and lethargic and her left side was weakening so much that I had to assist her with walking because her balance was being affected. A few days later we went for the MRI and then we were to see the oncologist right after.

It seemed to take forever sitting in that waiting room. Jean was with us this time, and Aleida stayed behind with my parents. Chantal was so tired that she lay against me and fell asleep. Finally, a nurse took her into a room where she could lie down. When the oncologist entered the room I knew it wasn't good just from the look on his face. He actually had to fight back tears trying to tell us the devastating news.

The original tumor, the one located in the thalamus, had grown quite large. It had increased from 1.4 to 4.2 centimeters and the other tumor in the mid-brain had grown from 1.0 to 1.6 centimeters. The oncologist informed Chantal that because of the swelling that she would have to go back on the Dexamethasone. Her first reaction was "Oh great, I'm gonna get fat again," and she began to cry. We all did. The oncologist advised to sleep with her head elevated. Now there was only one last resort. There was a new experimental drug called Irinotecan and when mixed with another drug, Avastin, it could possibly work.

Of course we were devastated and desperate. Wouldn't anyone be? In hindsight, we should have asked more questions. Questions like – how long have these drugs been tested? What are the results of the clinical trials? What are the adverse effects? But we were devastated. We knew Chantal's health was declining and our last hope was that these drugs could work.

The oncologist explained that the drugs could not be administered at the BC Cancer Agency as the Agency did not fund these experimental drugs. However, there was a doctor in Vancouver who had been working with them, and so we would have to travel to Vancouver.

Here's where some of the bureaucracy comes in. The biggest reason why the drug could not be administered at the BC Cancer Agency is not only because it was not funded, but also because only so many dollars are allotted per patient there. And it seemed that we had reached those allotted dollars. Even though millions of dollars are raised every year for cancer agencies like this one, there is still not enough money to cover the costs of drugs for the number of cancer patients. I'll get into this a little more later. Also, because the oncologist in Vancouver had been administering these drugs, the Cancer Agency people felt we should go there. Now we had to pack up Chantal, take the ferry, and go to this other hospital in Vancouver.

Wow, were we in for a surprise there.

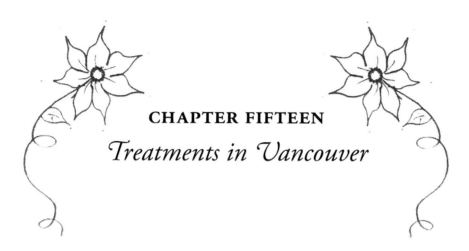

CHAPTER FIFTEEN
Treatments in Vancouver

CHANTAL WAS SCHEDULED FOR AN APPOINTMENT to see the oncologist in Vancouver for an assessment appointment and it was our understanding that she was to receive treatment right away. We knew we had to be there for a few days so we booked a hotel room close to the hospital.

We arrived at the hospital and waited for some time to see the oncologist. Chantal was very fatigued and becoming weaker on her left side so it was very hard on her to sit in a waiting room. Finally, we got a room where there was a bed and she could lie down. The oncologist arrived. He was hard to understand as he had a strong Slovak accent and he seemed very distracted. He would start to talk and then his beeper would go off. Out of the room he would go. He'd come back in, start to talk again, and now his cell rang. The entire appointment was like this; interrupted and sporadic. We were confused and didn't know what the hell was going on.

The oncologist grabbed Jean by the arm and took him to see a counselor. And the counselor got him to start filling out forms – I didn't even know where he went. All I could do was stand there and say, "What the fuck just happened here?"

Jean returned to the room and told us that the counselor had explained to him what the treatment drugs would be, how and when they'd be administered, and that we could try to get the drug manufacturer to cover the costs. (Incidentally, this trillion-dollar corporation would not.) Then we were told that we had to go across the street to the pharmacy to get the drugs for her first treatment for the next day.

We thought it was odd. Why would *we* have to go and pick up these drugs for chemotherapy especially when they were going to be administered in a hospital? But off we went, thinking that we were just "picking up" these drugs just like we had at the BC Cancer Agency. So I talked to the pharmacist and gave her the prescription and we waited in the pharmacy for it to be filled. We were then told it was ready.

There were four drugs:

Avastin: $2276.96

Irinotecan: $1285.70

Kytril: $136.86

Stemetil: $13.00

TOTAL: $3712.47

As I took the bag and was ready to walk away, the pharmacist said, "That will be $3712.47."

W*HAT????* "Uh…" I explained that I had not been expecting to be paying for these drugs. NO ONE had indicated that we had to pay. We couldn't afford to pay! At this point we were nearly tapped out. So I said to the pharmacist, "If I can't pay for these right now, does that mean my daughter doesn't get treatment tomorrow?"

And her sad face said a soft-spoken, "Yes."

I freaked. And so did Jean. We panicked as to what to do next until I managed to calm myself down to try to think of what to do. I called one of my brothers, and crying on the phone, freaking out, I attempted to tell him what was going on, After all of that, he simply put it on his credit card. What a savior to us. Incidentally, he has never asked for any of the money back as it was something he was doing for Chantal.

We returned to our hotel room confused, stressed, and exhausted. It was a very trying day.

The next day, we returned to the hospital for Chantal's first treatment with these experimental and very expensive drugs, which had to be administered intravenously. As we walked into the large treatment room, I couldn't believe how many people were in there, all hooked up and receiving chemotherapy treatment. It was unreal to me and I couldn't understand it. All I could think was, *What is this world coming to that all these people are sick with cancer and are here, hooked up to machines and having chemicals pumped into their bodies? And* now, my daughter had to do the same. It saddened me even more.

We were informed that Chantal would have to return every two weeks for treatment and that we would have to purchase the drugs each time at a cost of approximately $4000 every two weeks. They were not covered by the BC Cancer Agency or by Jean's or my health benefits. We didn't know what we were going to do.

CHAPTER SIXTEEN
Chemotherapy Drugs and the Medical System

WHEN CHANTAL FIRST BEGAN CHEMOTHERAPY IN August of 2006, it had been in pill form. And with all the other drugs she'd been prescribed, it felt like we had a small pharmacy at home. We were fortunate that most of the drug costs were covered by the BC Cancer Agency and partially by our health benefits, and we'd only had to pay a small portion.

When it came time for her treatments at the Lion's Gate Hospital in Vancouver with the Irinotecan (also known as Temozolomide) we were not so lucky. I called the company through which I got my health benefits and I was informed that neither Irinotecan nor Avastin were covered because it showed that the hospital was supposed to cover the costs. It was suggested that perhaps we should try to get some provincial funding. I asked if the company would provide a letter stating that they did not cover the drug costs. I hoped that I could forward it to Jean's health benefit company to see if they would cover them.

Jean's plan indicated the same information.

The rep at my health benefit company asked if the drugs were administered in a clinic separate from the hospital. When I said they were administered in a hospital, she stated that I could contact the company that makes Avastin to see if they could help. So I contacted the company and they informed me that if we were to go to a private infusion clinic that the drug would be covered 100% with no deductible or maximums. They also said that we could use our health benefit drug card at the clinic to pay for the Avastin (after some lengthy paperwork between the doctor and the clinic had been filled out). Except there was a catch – a few in fact. First, they would not cover the other drug, Irinotecan, because it is considered a cytotoxic drug. It can only be administered in a hospital because it is a hospital prescription drug, which our government is supposed to be covering. Avastin is not cytotoxic and can be administered in a private infusion clinic. Cytotoxic drugs can prevent the rapid growth and division of cancer cells. But their side effects are alarming even to the hospital workers who handle them. Google it.

It was discussed that we could take her to a private clinic in Vancouver to have the Avastin administered, (which I Google-mapped would be at least forty-five minute to an hour's drive to the Lion's Gate Hospital). Then we'd have to go to the Lion's Gate Hospital to have the Irinotecan administered. Wasn't going to work. Secondly, at the private infusion clinic, the Avastin was administered by advanced cardiac life support nurses NOT chemotherapy nurses.

I couldn't believe the information I was being given and I was confused as to what to do. So I called the oncologist at the BC Cancer Agency, asked him if he had ever heard of these types of clinics and if we were to go this route, what would happen with Chantal's care. He informed me that he had never heard of these clinics and was surprised that our benefit plans were not covering the drugs. Okay… now what the hell to do?

I could not believe that there were private infusion clinics available. I had never heard of this before. Private clinics in Canada? What was up with our health system? What was going on between the health benefit plan company and the pharmaceutical companies?

Jean worked at the local hospital in Duncan – a two-minute drive from where we lived. One day, he told the pharmacist or one of the nurses there that we had to go to Vancouver for treatments because the drugs were only administered there. The nurse said that she couldn't believe that we were going all the way to Vancouver when the drugs could be administered right at the hospital in Duncan.

Why had we not been told that in the first place by the people in Victoria or in Vancouver? We had already gone to Vancouver twice and we were not looking forward to any more trips as they were so hard on Chantal. The drive to the ferry was forty-five minutes, wait time at the ferry was anywhere from a half-hour to an hour (on each side), and the drive to the hospital in Vancouver was at least thirty minutes. The chemo nurse checked into it, and sure enough we could bring Chantal right there to the Duncan hospital and have her treatments there.

After the first treatment, we were given a bill and it was only $2495.45 Because it was so much less than it had been in Vancouver we thought that there must be an error. Jean asked the pharmacist why it was cheaper and he was informed that hospitals will get together to have more buying power and can therefore purchase the drugs at a cheaper rate from the pharmaceutical companies.

Why did we have to find this out as we went along? Why can't this kind of information be up front right from the beginning, so that families like ours do not have to be jacked around? Especially having been sent to Vancouver when we could have gone right to our local hospital only five minutes away.

As I mentioned earlier, I chucked out a lot of the medical receipts and notes from this time, but in writing this I did find a few things. I have a medical report from the oncologist and as I read it I could not recall it from back when Chantal's health really started to fail. In the oncologist's report, it states that there were many treatments available but that the likelihood of response at this time was low. It also says, "…the most interesting treatment option prior to this point is a combination of Avastin and Irinotecan. There have been several phase II trials published showing impressive response rates and progressive free survival in recurrent glioblastoma multiforme." Something that the oncologist had said at Chantal's appointment when we found out that the tumors had grown was that the Oncologists' Association had just had a big conference in San Francisco and it was discussed there that this drug combination was the latest and greatest in treatment options.

After Chantal started the treatment of these two drugs combined, I began my own research. I found that the clinical trials had only been done on a hundred people over a six-month to two-year period and that the patients experienced many side effects, as Chantal did. And that survival rate was zero. To me, that more or less said: Let's keep the patients alive a little longer and put them through hell while we're at it.

What do you do?

CHAPTER SEVENTEEN

Where Is the Money Going to Come From?

APPROXIMATELY $4000 EVERY TWO WEEKS FOR chemotherapy drugs – drugs not covered by any health plan or cancer agency. We didn't know what we were going to do. Because our home was so new, we didn't have enough equity to borrow from. Jean had money in a pension plan from a previous job, so with assistance from our investors' group advisor, Jean was able to access some money from this. As I implied earlier, we were tapped out. We already had a few credit cards that were maxed out and our line of credit was already quite high from paying for the drugs. And because I wasn't working, we couldn't access any more credit. The bank gave us a few extensions on our mortgage payment and vehicle payment but that was it. Nothing more could be done. Combining my lost income with the cost of the drugs amounted to just almost $5000…every – two – weeks.

We confided in our families and friends as to the cost of the treatment drugs and that we didn't know what we were going to do. I was on a leave of absence from work, and therefore I had no income so we were totally reliant on Jean's, which was not huge. And then, fundraisers started to happen. Oh my God! We couldn't believe the involvement and the love and care that went into these fundraisers to help us. Even though we now lived on Vancouver Island, our friends and family back home in Peace River, Alberta were putting together fundraisers in the community. One of my closest and best friends, Cara, approached a local festival to help raise money and every person working the festival who usually got an honorarium, donated his or her money to our cause. Chantal's friends Colleen and Shivon organized a community bottle drive. People were invited to bring in their bottles to the bottle depot and the money was then donated to our cause. My mother-in-law, Marie organized a bottle drive in the community of Jean Cote and surrounding area. People constantly dropped off bottles to their farm and she and my father-in-law and many of Jean's siblings and their families also helped in the sorting and delivering of the bottles to the bottle depot. Cara, along with my sister Shauna, sister-in-law Debe, and Chantal's friend Colleen starting organizing a dance with a silent auction. Friends who are musicians volunteered to provide the entertainment, silent auction items were donated left and right from the business community, and the weekend even grew into a pancake breakfast the next day. More friends and my family members were involved to help make the weekend a huge success. People were even handing money to my family members and saying, "Here take it"! The weekend brought in over $37,000!!! And at Jean's place of work, a hot dog/hamburger sale during a noon hour brought in $6000!!

Checks started coming in the mail from relatives and friends. It seemed every day that I stopped at the mail box there was another check in the mail. Because we lived so far away from family and friends, Jean had created a web page called "Supporting Chantal" where people could post words of encouragement for Chantal and our family. He added a PayPal account to it so people could also donate online. And money started coming that way too. Because I was well known in my hometown community, it was even mentioned on the local radio station and strangers from Peace River and in the listening area began donating. It was unbelievable to us how much love and support was being provided to us in our time of need. Not hundreds of dollars but thousands of dollars were being donated privately or through fundraisers. We were so overwhelmed by this outpouring of love and support and we are forever grateful to everyone who contributed.

CHAPTER EIGHTEEN
A Desperate Mother

CHANTAL'S HEALTH WAS FAILING AND FAILING fast. It seemed like every day her left side weakened more and more. Walking became more difficult and for her to get anywhere we had to get a wheelchair. Our house was three levels; with the living room and kitchen on the main floor and the bedrooms upstairs. In order for Chantal to get to her bedroom, we tried putting her on a chair that Jean and I would carry upstairs. But that became very hard on us so we had to purchase and install a chair lift. We didn't have walk-in showers, only tubs, and she could not lift her leg to get into the tub to have a shower or a bath. So we rented a lift to get her in and out of the tub. Thank goodness for all the fundraisers or else we would never have been able to afford these items. It's unbelievable to me how expensive assistive medical devices are. It's friggin' robbery!!

Early after Chantal's diagnosis, I started to research how food can affect our health. Holy shit! I could write a book just about nutrition and what is happening to our food on this planet.

Sugar is the enemy. Yes, there are the natural fruit sugars but I'm talking about all the "fake" sugars that are found in our foods today. What it boils down to is that we should eat our fruits, vegetables, proteins, and whole grains and even then you have to be careful what is in our foods – antibiotics, chemicals sprayed on the vegetables and fruits, chemicals used to strip grains. Anything boxed, canned, or jarred is ALL full of sugar and chemicals. Why do these types of foods taste so good? Processed sugars and chemicals. And sugar feeds cancer cells. Because we lived on Vancouver Island we were fortunate enough to have many organic farms around us where I could purchase fruits and vegetables that were not sprayed and meat from farms that did not use antibiotics. Again, I could write an entire book about what is in our foods and why organic is so much better. Some people don't believe that it is, but I would like you to think about this – think of farms in the old days. Cows grazed freely in the pastures and ate grass, and vegetables were grown in gardens where no chemicals were used to kill the weeds. Grains were grown in open fields and no chemicals were sprayed on them either. We have become a chemical and drug-dependent society and it's killing us slowly.

I read a lot of books and researched on the Internet to find healthy recipes. To reduce the swelling caused by the edema around the tumors in her brain, Chantal was back on Dexamethasone, and as before, her appetite increased immensely. I was constantly preparing food for her and I wanted it to be as healthy as possible. Of course, she didn't like it at first as all the "good stuff" was taken out of her diet. I had to tell her repeatedly that I was removing sugar from her diet so that it didn't feed the cancer cells.

Because of the fundraising dollars coming in, I was able to purchase a Vita-Mix blender. These blenders cost approximately $400 but you have them for a lifetime of healthy eating. In my mind, every household should have one. I was able to make homemade frozen desserts, soups, dressings, sauces – all using fruits, vegetables and herbs, and natural ingredients. Chantal loved her bread but I at least tried to keep that to a minimum, and there was a wonderful organic bakery that we had access to.

Because we weren't sure if the drugs were going to work I also started researching natural remedies. I was constantly busy. Taking care of Chantal was now becoming more and more demanding, but I wanted to try anything and everything that I could possibly do to keep her alive.

Once again, because we lived on Vancouver Island, we had access to many different types of natural remedies and therapies. I would find holistic practitioners, take Chantal to them for an assessment, and decide if that was an option. But even taking her out was starting to become a lot of work as she was pretty much confined to a wheel-chair. I would have to lift her from her wheelchair, put her in the vehicle, and then take her out of the vehicle and into the wheelchair. She was becoming heavier again because of the Dexamethasone and it was getting more difficult for me to lift her. But I was in constant panic mode. I didn't care about myself – all I cared about was trying to get my daughter better. There was no way I was giving up. This was my child who I loved more than anything and I was bound and determined to go to any lengths for her survival.

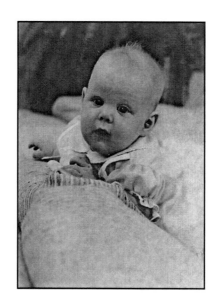

CHANTAL AT 3 MONTHS

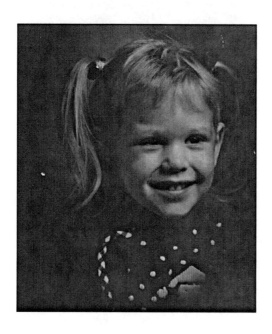

CHANTAL AGE 2 YRS

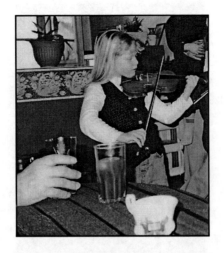

CHANTAL PLAYING THE VIOLIN

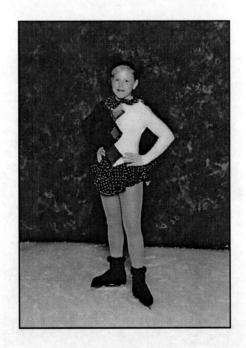

CHANTAL FIGURE SKATING

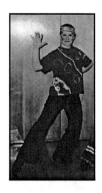

CHANTAL HIP HOP DANCE

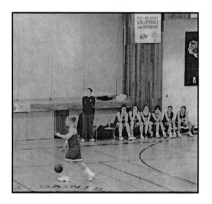

CHANTAL PLAYING BASKETBALL

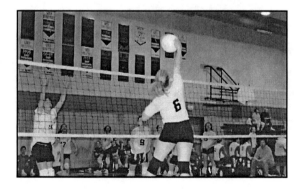

PLAYING VOLLEYBALL

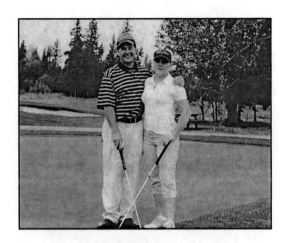

WITH UNCLE DAVE

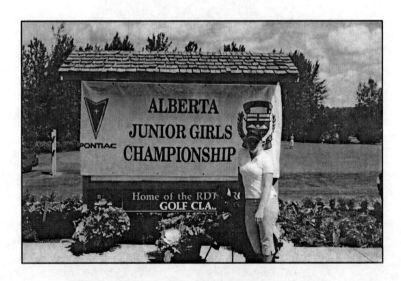

HER FIRST PROVINCIAL GOLF TOURNAMENT

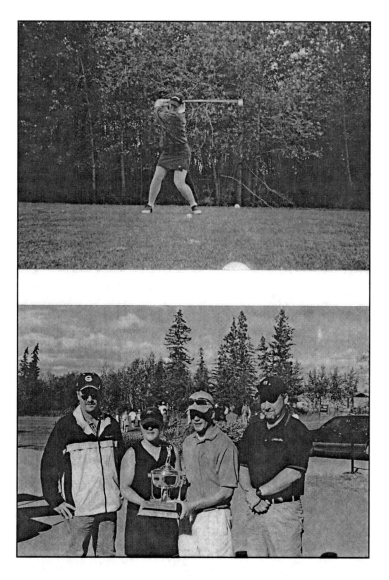

MIGHTY PEACE JUNIOR CHAMPIONSHIP

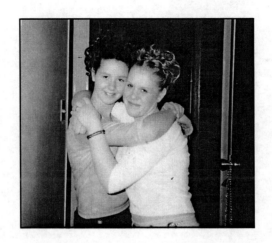

WITH CARLEE. CHANTAL DONE THEIR HAIR FOR GRADE 9 DANCE

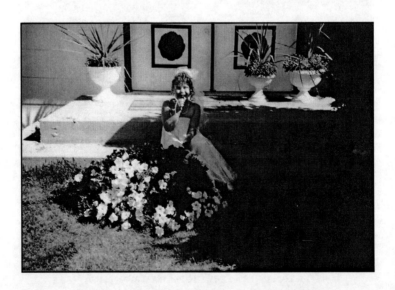

CHANTAL DRESSED ALEIDA AS A LITTLE BRIDE

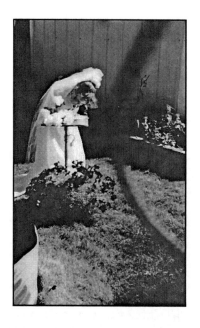

AFTER CHANTAL PERFORMED THE WEDDING CEREMONY

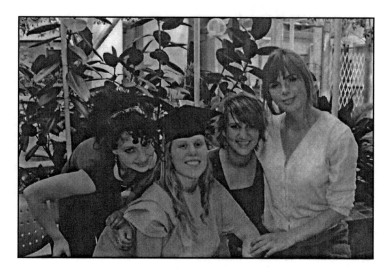

A VISIT FROM EMMA , SHIVON AND MICHELLE AT UOFA HOSPITAL

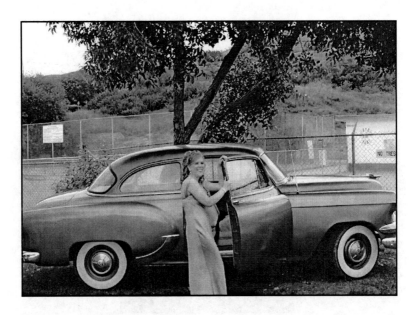

CHANTAL'S PRIVATE GRAD PARTY

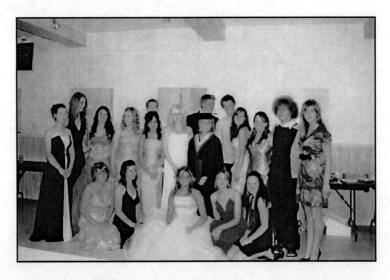

HER FRIENDS DRESSED UP AGAIN FOR HER PRIVATE GRAD PARTY

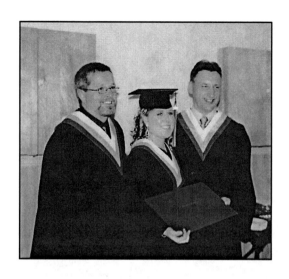

CHANTAL BEING PRESENTED WITH HIGH SCHOOL DIPLOMA BY
PRINCIPAL AND VICE PRINCIPAL AT PRIVATE GRAD PARTY

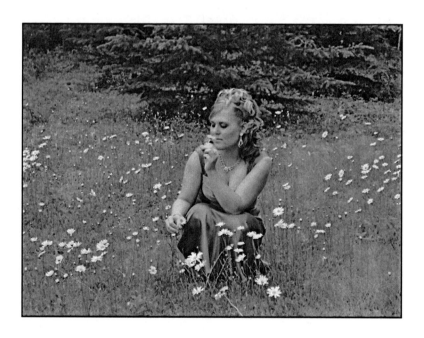

ON THE PRIVATE PARTY GRAD DAY.

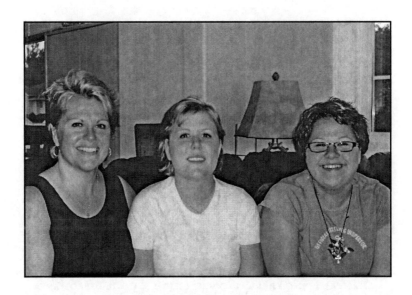

OUR HAIR CUTS

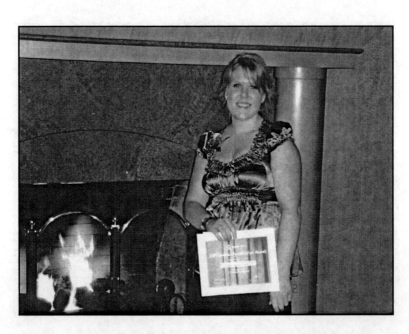

CHANTAL'S $2500 SCHOLARSHIP TOWARDS UNIVERSITY

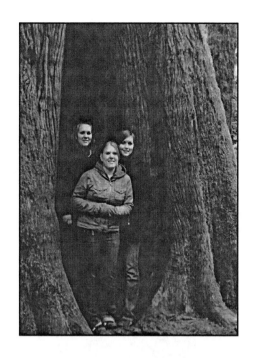

MEGAN, AMANDA CAME TO VISIT. THIS IS IN
CATHEDRAL GROVE ON VANCOUVER ISLAND

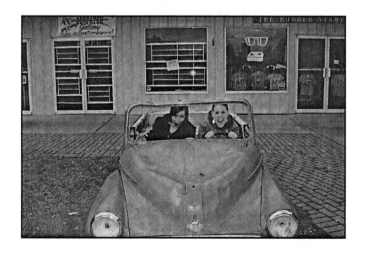

AMANDA AND CHANTAL GOOFING AROUND IN COOMBS, BC

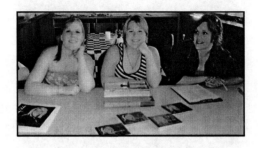

CHANTAL, ALEIDA AND JENNIFER SELLING
CD'S AT MY CD RELEASE PARTY

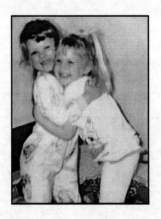

MEGAN AND CHANTAL CHILDHOOD FRIENDS.
MANY PEOPLE THOUGHT THEY WERE TWINS

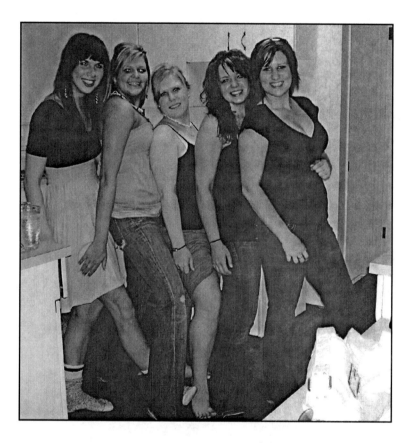

L–R MICHELLE, ASHLEA, CHANTAL, COLLEEN AND SHIVON

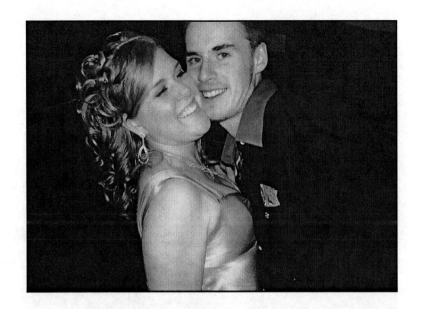

CHANTAL AND MATT

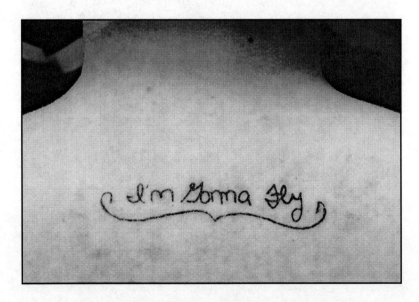

**TATTOO THAT CHANTAL'S FRIENDS AND ALEIDA
GOT ON CHANTAL'S BIRTHDAY**

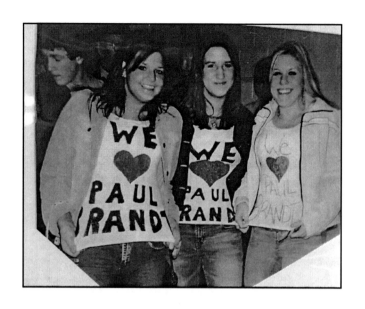

ASHLEA, SHIVON AND CHANTAL AT A PAUL BRANDT CONCERT

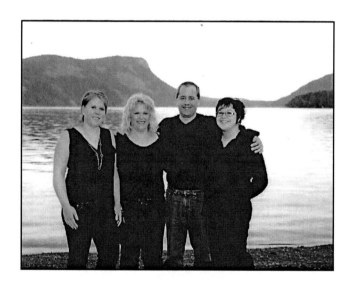

OUR LAST FAMILY PHOTO TAKEN IN MAPLE BAY, BC

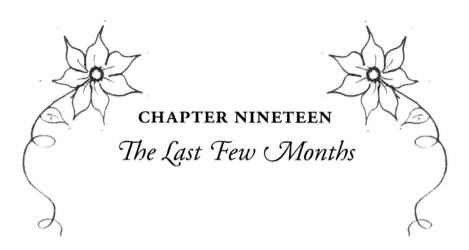

CHAPTER NINETEEN
The Last Few Months

CHANTAL'S HEALTH CONTINUED TO DECLINE AND the more it declined, the more desperate I became to do anything to save her life.

The chemotherapy drug combination of Avastin and Irinotecan was showing its side effects. Chantal was sleeping a lot and she had started to experience unbearable leg pain. The pain was so bad it made her cry and yell out how much it hurt. It was really getting hard to watch my poor child go through so much. Because of the leg pain, I took her into the hospital to have her checked. There was swelling around one knee and the emergency doctor thought she might have water on the knee, so he had to insert this huge needle into her knee, and this was also very painful for her. There was such a scared look on her face before he inserted the needle. She had been brave before about needles, but now she was tired of being poked and prodded and so tired of the pain that she just didn't want it any more. I almost yelled at the doctor to STOP! I couldn't take it anymore either. The result was that we learned there was no water on the knee and the swelling was determined to be a side effect from the treatments. So guess what. More medication was prescribed. Morphine. Yeah, let's add another drug to the mix. But I know the pain was unbearable for her and every time the leg pain would hit a morphine pill was taken.

Chantal had blood tests on a regular basis to watch her platelets and her white blood cell count. At a chemo treatment appointment in July (when we were still going to Vancouver), an oncologist checked her blood test results, which indicated that her platelets and white blood cells were too low for a full treatment. Because of this, a full dose of Avastin but just a hint of Irinotecan was administered. Because we had by then found out that the treatments could be done in Duncan, we asked the oncologist to have Chantal's treatments transferred to the Duncan hospital. He made a phone call and it was done. Thank goodness we didn't have to travel back and forth to Vancouver any more. Oh, and another drug had to be administered to help rebuild Chantal's white blood cell count. One shot of Neulasta (a growth factor stimulator that had to be administered by a doctor) needed to be given twenty-four to forty-eight hours after this chemo treatment. This was purchased at our local drug store and was eighty percent covered by my extended health plan. Thank goodness, as it was $2400. Also, there was another drug prescribed called Naprosyn, an anti-inflammatory, because there could be bone pain, which is a side effect of the Neulasta. It never ended.

Some of Chantal's long-time girlfriends, Shivon and Colleen came for a visit and it gave her some uplifted spirits. It was so good that her friends could be there to laugh and joke with her. While they visited, they saw what Chantal was going through and provided comfort and support to both of us. When they left, they each left a letter for Chantal to read and their words of encouragement and love were incredible. I still have these letters.

Chantal also received gifts of childhood memories from other long-time girlfriends Ashlea and Megan who were unable to come out at that time. Megan made her an album from their childhood and Ashlea made a collage of pictures of all their good times in a huge frame.

Love, cards, letters of support, and other gifts were pouring in from friends and relatives. All of them provided words of encouragement suggesting, "You'll get through this."

Chantal's boyfriend, Matthew had continued to stay by her side all through this. He was there when she ended up in the U of A Hospital in Edmonton right through until now. He had been dealing with everything quite well, but as her health declined further it was getting more and more difficult for him to watch her go through this.

August came and it was getting even harder for Chantal to handle the treatments. While receiving them, she was in a comfy recliner, a lift chair that had been loaned to us by the parents of one of Jean's co-workers, but she would always have to get out and go to the washroom because the treatment made her have to urinate. She could no longer walk on her own, but the need to urinate was intense and urgent so it became even more difficult to receive the treatments. As she was lying there, all of a sudden she would say, "I have to pee and now!" Trying to get her out of the recliner, into the wheelchair, over to the bathroom, and then on the toilet was quite an episode. And this of course, started to upset her greatly.

We still had some visitors coming and going and Chantal, Jean, Aleida, and I were happy that people took the time to come out and see us and provide some support.

I continued to feed Chantal and the rest of the family a healthy diet. I was constantly researching about food and alternate therapies and I was in a constant mode of taking care of Chantal.

After researching different alternate therapies, we found a couple of ladies who helped us out. One provided Reiki therapy and Ionic Foot Detox to help with the side effects of the chemotherapy, and the other provided information about how to remove sugar from the diet and put healthy vitamins in the body.

For a body to be healthy, it must be in an alkaline state. Because of all the chemicals that had been put into Chantal's body, a pH test showed that she was very acidic. An acidic body is a sick body – disease thrives in an acidic body. The Ionic Foot Detox helped to draw out the toxins left over from the chemotherapy drugs. The Reiki was done for Chantal's emotional state, to help clear her mind from any emotional situations – past or present. The mind and body are incredible and both need to be clear to be in a healthy state.

Vitamins, in their purest state, are vital in today's environment. Our foods are laced with chemicals and many are now genetically modified so that food cannot provide the essential vitamins that our bodies need. But we found a lady (with credentials), who provided guidance on healthy eating and which vitamins to take.

By September, the chemotherapy was really wearing down Chantal. The leg pain was still happening and we couldn't keep feeding her morphine. Chantal, Jean, and I discussed what to do and we decided that she needed a rest from the chemotherapy treatments. We met with the oncologist in the Duncan hospital, told him our decision, and he honored it.

By mid-September, Chantal started losing even more control of certain body functions. Her bladder became very weak, and I was constantly changing her bed sheets as accidents started to happen. Her nights consisted of interrupted sleep, so I would sleep beside her, either on her bed or on the floor of her bedroom. She was deteriorating in front of my eyes, but we continued to pray to our guardian angels to please help her become well.

I was becoming extremely exhausted and was running on little energy, but I had to keep going. Somehow I found the strength, but it was getting more and more difficult to take her out of bed and move her downstairs. Having the chair lift installed helped immensely. I would help her out of bed, put her in the wheelchair, wheel her over to the chairlift, and help her into that. The chairlift went down one flight of stairs and then I had to move her to the next chair lift for the second set of stairs, leave her on the chair lift, get the wheelchair, and then transfer her into the wheelchair.

We were now confined to the house. It was impossible to take her out anywhere because of her urinary incontinence and because she was too difficult to move. Jean continued to work and Aleida had just started her grade eleven year, so they were gone during the day but when they came home they helped with cooking supper and going out to get groceries and supplies. We could no longer go out for Reiki treatments.

By the end of the month I was so exhausted that I called up my mom and dad and asked if they could come out to help me. I had to finally admit that I couldn't do this by myself anymore. They were able to come out the week before Thanksgiving to stay for a few weeks or more.

Chantal continued to deteriorate. She was now losing control of her bowels as well as her bladder. As much as I hated to do it, I had to put her in Depends. I was now changing my twenty-year-old daughter's diapers. She never said anything, but I knew she hated it. Hated it with a passion. It was even getting too difficult to continue to move her from her room to the main floor so I made a bed on the couch.

One night, I had Chantal downstairs in the living room and we were watching TV. My mom and dad were sitting at the dining room table, and I had gotten up off the couch to go get something in the kitchen. Jean was working an evening shift and Aleida was working at her part-time job. As I walked back, Chantal's head started to rotate to the left and it looked weird – like it was happening involuntarily. I ran to her and asked her if she knew what was happening. She couldn't answer me and then she began vomiting. I freaked out and started to panic. I didn't want this to happen. This wasn't supposed to be happening. She was supposed to be getting better! I knew this was not good, so I called Jean and told him that he had to come home. He only had an hour left in his shift, but he was able to get a hold of his boss and come home. We then called the ambulance.

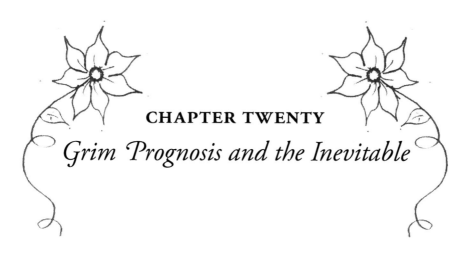

CHAPTER TWENTY
Grim Prognosis and the Inevitable

CHANTAL HAD A SEIZURE AND IT was the beginning of more. The emergency doctor examined her and then they did a CT scan to get a picture of what was happening. The tumors were causing even more pressure and edema was quite apparent, therefore the resulting seizures. We had not done any chemotherapy for almost two months at this point and there was nothing more that could be done. But I still was not ready to give up. Chantal continued to have mini-seizures while in the hospital and the hospital staff were keeping her comfortable. The doctors painted a grim picture, but I didn't want to accept it. To me, this still was not going to happen. I was not going to let my daughter die!! And to top things off, we received a phone call from one of my cousins telling us that my dad's brother had passed away.

They had a lady come in from Hospice to talk to us about keeping Chantal comfortable in the hospital, but I wouldn't have it. It was Friday and Thanksgiving weekend. My mom was there and Chantal was looking forward to having Grandma's cabbage rolls. So we took her home, got her up to her bedroom, and made her comfortable. Jean and my mom and dad kept her company in her room by playing a lot of crib. The mini-seizures continued and we continued to pray.

We took turns sitting with Chantal, and my friend Jen and Chantal's boyfriend Matthew came and sat with her as well. By Monday night around eleven p.m., the seizures had become so frequent and intense we had to take her back to the hospital. Once again, we called the ambulance and it just so happened it was the same paramedics. My parents and Aleida were sleeping so we woke them up to tell them we were taking Chantal to the hospital.

The end was very near. Chantal was no longer conscious and therefore could not verbalize. Her heart was racing and it was the only thing keeping her alive. The attending doctor said it was only a matter of time.

NO!!!!!! THIS WAS NOT HAPPENING!! THIS WAS NOT SUPPOSED TO HAPPEN!!! WE PRAYED!! WE THOUGHT POSITIVE THOUGHTS!!

My parents and Aleida arrived early in the morning and when they walked in we told them what the doctor had said. We all fell apart.

They moved Chantal from emergency up to a private room. Jean and my parents made calls to family to tell them the news.

A bunch of family members decided to make the trip out to be with us. Even my father-in-law, who had never been on a plane before, flew out to be with us.

It was Wednesday and the family had arrived. Even one of Chantal's friends since childhood, Brandyn, came out to be with us. So for two days, Chantal was surrounded by her family and friends. We prayed, we talked to her, and they helped support us. Jean, Aleida, and I were not leaving. The nurses got us a cot so we could sleep in Chantal's room. One of us would sleep while the other sat with Chantal. Jean slept on the floor a lot if someone else was using the cot. Chantal was in that room, Room 206, for about two days then she was moved to a another room, Room 214, on the same floor but in another wing.

I begged her to wake up. I wanted her to wake up!! I wanted this nightmare to be over and for her to be well again!!

During that time, Chantal's lungs kept filling up with fluid, and the nurses would have to come in and use an instrument to suck the fluid out. They told us that at this point the only thing keeping her alive was her strong heart.

Friday, October 17th just before eight a.m., Jean and I went out the hallway. We had finally accepted that this was the end and that it was time for us to tell her that it was okay for her to go – that she no longer had to suffer. Jean said that he just needed to go to the washroom to freshen up and that when he came back we would tell her. I went back into the room, sat beside her, and constantly stroked her body. They say that people's souls leave their bodies long before their bodies die. Well, Chantal must have been in that hallway listening to us because her heart rate started to drop and quickly. The nurses came in and as she was slipping away, Jean came into the room as well.

Even though we had made that decision, it was still too real to accept. As her heart continued to slow, I yelled NO!!!!! And then... her heart stopped and she was gone. There lay her body. Still. My whole body felt weak and I cried uncontrollably. What I had been trying so hard to prevent from happening had just happened, and there was nothing more I could do. Chantal's heart had stopped and mine was broken. Forever.

Chantal was surrounded by some of the people she loved the most. Me, Jean, Aleida, my parents Ray and Mary, my sister Karen, my sister Shauna, my brother David and his wife Jana, my brother Gary and his wife Debe, Jean's parents Gerard and Marie, his sister Sylvia and husband Hervey, my friend Jennifer and her son Matthew (Chantal's boyfriend), Brandyn, and Jean's Aunt Fran and Uncle Tony.

I stood by her bedside for some time. I didn't want to leave. This just didn't happen. What do you mean I have to leave my daughter's body here? What do you mean I can't take her home? What am I going to do without my baby girl?

I was numb. We had to sign papers and I didn't even remember what I was signing. Chantal had expressed at some time in her life that she wanted to be an organ donor. But because of the cancer, all that could be donated were her eyes. So she was able to give the gift to sight to someone else.

It was some time later, I don't know how long, and everyone else was hungry and wanted to go out for breakfast. I had not eaten very well in days, and nobody else had really had a decent meal in a few days either. I followed along, still numb, thinking, *What the hell am I doing going out for breakfast? My* daughter had just died. I didn't want to be there. I wanted to go home. So finally, eating was done and we went home. I ran up to Chantal's room, fell on her bed, and cried uncontrollably. I think I was in hysterics. My parents came in, sat me up, and sat on either side of me. They held me and we all cried.

This was real. My daughter was dead and was never coming home again.

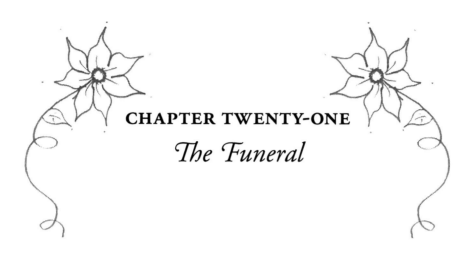

CHAPTER TWENTY-ONE
The Funeral

WHY IS IT THAT FUNERALS HAVE to happen so fast? A person is numb. Your loved one has just passed away and now you have to make funeral arrangements? All the decisions you have to make while you can't think straight!

Because all our long-time friends and family were in Peace River and area, we decided to have the funeral in Peace River. We didn't want a church funeral (Chantal had disliked church funerals and so did Jean and I), so we decided to book the school gym where Chantal went to school. We knew it was going to be a large funeral and we'd need the space. Then we had to make arrangements for her body to be transported from Duncan to Peace River, and we had to book flights for ourselves.

It was hard to pack a bag and leave the house. But in my numbness I was able to go through the motions as we all were.

Once we got to Peace River we had to visit the funeral home. The funeral home had been in the same place since I was kid and I'd always hated driving by there. Death always scared me and I never wanted to have to go into that place. And here I was, going in to make funeral arrangements for my daughter.

We decided that we would rent a casket so that family and friends who wanted to see Chantal's body one last time could have the option to do so. I wanted to see her again. All I could think about was her body being transported in some cold case from funeral home to airport, and airport to funeral home, and I wasn't there.

We asked my sisters Shauna and Karen to read the eulogy and Chantal's lifetime friends to read stories about their "times" with Chantal. Of course we had asked some of her closest guy friends and a few of her favorite cousins to be the pallbearers. A lifelong friend of the family was a minister, so we asked her to officiate at the service and to keep it non-denominational. Flowers for the casket were Chantal's favorites – gerbera daisies and lilies, and the colors were teal-blue mixed with white. We had a beautiful picture of Chantal sitting amongst Shasta daisies, which had been taken before her graduation party, and we had it enlarged, framed, and displayed at the service. Beside it was a large candle that we still burn every year on the anniversary of her passing. We wanted the service to be about Chantal – not God or any religion, because to me that's not what it's about. It's about the person we are mourning.

Chantal's friends got together and created a slide presentation – photos and video of Chantal with friends and family doing some of her favorite activities. We also included a clip of a video that I had recorded while she was golfing with some friends – she had made a forty-foot put and was pretty impressed with herself. It showed Chantal's character. The music was taken care of by my girlies Cara and Shelley, along with some of Chantal's teachers, Joanne and Nicola. About two years before, prior to Chantal being diagnosed, I had discovered a beautiful song, "I Will See You Again" by Rhonda Vincent and I asked the girls to sing it.

The entire time we were making all these preparations, I was still numb. I kept thinking: *What the hell am I doing? What am I arranging? This isn't real!* And then came the day of the service. Jean, Aleida, and I and all the immediate family and closest friends were in a separate room – waiting. Waiting to make that dreaded entrance into the gym following the casket. I had watched so many others and done it a few times myself for my grandparents, but this was different. Still, I was in and out of reality and a dream world. Then it was time for the private viewing. I so badly wanted to see her again. At any other funeral, I NEVER go to the body because I want to remember people alive – not dead. And here I was, looking at my daughter's cold, dead body. She had puffed up so much from all the drugs and the edema, I just kept saying, "It doesn't look like her." I hated how she looked. Her beautiful face and body were all bloated up. That wasn't her. I did not want to accept that this was really happening.

I guess it was a beautiful service with about seven hundred people in attendance. Everyone did such a great job and the music was perfect but…I don't remember most of it. I cried and I cried and I cried and I cried. All I wanted to do was run to the casket, open it up and yell, "Get up!!!!! Let's get the hell out of here!!!!" But it wasn't to be so. Everyone said it was a beautiful service and that they loved how it was all about Chantal. Exactly what I wanted.

I don't like graveyards so we had decided to have Chantal's body cremated, and after the service was over we followed her casket to the hearse. As they loaded her body into it I finally realized, this is it! This is my final goodbye! OH MY GOD!! I will never see her again. I could feel myself falling to my knees but my mother was beside me and held me up. I was crumbling physically and emotionally. I had nothing left.

As we walked back inside the school, I was constantly hugged, again and again. Now I know people just don't know what to say and I want to say here, if you don't know what to say, please just be silent or say, "I don't know what to say," and then a hug will be all that is needed. I don't know how many times I heard, "She's in a better place" or "God will take care of her." NO!! For me, she was not in a better place! A better place was with me! And I would take care of her! Not God! All I wanted to do was fall down and fall apart. But I couldn't because so many people wanted to express their sadness and sympathy. Of course there was the luncheon and then afterwards we had rented another facility for all the relatives and friends to gather. After a few hours, I just wanted to hide. I was done.

A few days later, we returned to the funeral home to pick out an urn and we also picked out jewelry that you can place ashes into. I chose a heart, Jean chose a cross, Aleida and my mom and mother-in-law chose angels and for the grandpas they each chose a small urn.

Jean and I were able to wear the jewelry for a little while, but we both found that it was too heavy on our hearts. And to this day, I still cannot wear any heavy pendants over my heart. The rest of Chantal's ashes were placed into a beautiful, teal-blue urn with doves.

It was over. Everything had come to an end and I was devastated.

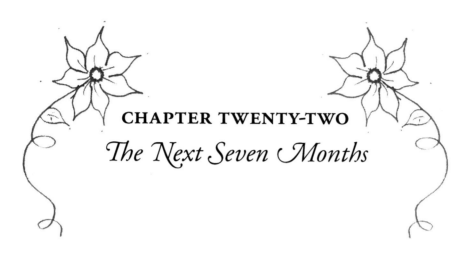

CHAPTER TWENTY-TWO
The Next Seven Months

WE RETURNED TO OUR HOME IN Duncan and all was quiet. I immediately ran up to Chantal's room, looked around, lay on her bed and sobbed. Her smell was still in her bed sheets and blankets, and all I could do was breathe in her scent. It was all I had left of her.

Every day, I would get up, go in her bedroom, bawl my eyes out, and sometimes yell out, "WHY?? WHY MY CHILD??" And sometimes it was a scream. I was so heartbroken and angry. What had I done to deserve this? What had Chantal done to deserve this? This wasn't fair!!! Why was my heart being ripped out like this? I actually felt pain in my chest because my heart was so broken.

Jean took time off work for approximately two and half months and Aleida stayed home from school for a few weeks. I was able to obtain long-term disability through my extended health benefits. We walked around like zombies.

Jean removed the medical assistive devices we had rented – the bathtub lift, the portable potty in her bedroom, and the wheelchair. The chair lift remained for a few days, but then Jean took it down as it was too much of a reminder of how bad Chantal's condition had been. We'd had to purchase the stair lift and it was difficult to try and sell it, so we stored it in the garage until we could get rid of it.

After bawling my eyes out in Chantal's room, I would proceed downstairs, and still in my pajamas, sit on the couch and watch TV all day long. I showered once in a while, but I wouldn't do my hair or make up. What was the point? I didn't want to go anywhere and I cried every day. I didn't even go outside. I should have gone for walks as we had beautiful walking trails right outside our door and my poor dog Presley sure needed to get out, but I didn't care. After Jean returned to work and Aleida was in school, Presley was my companion during the day. We both lay on the couch.

I can't remember if I would go out to get groceries. I think Jean and Aleida were taking care of that and making meals. My grief was starting to affect my marriage and my relationship with my other daughter, Aleida, but I had no concept that I was leaving them out. One day, during one of my crying fits in Chantal's bedroom, Jean came in and sat beside me and cried too. But then he said to me, "I want my wife back."

This made me really angry and I yelled at him, "You can't! I don't have my daughter!!" and he left the room. We were there to comfort one another, but there was no intimacy for about a year.

Aleida's bedroom was right beside Chantal's and many times she had to listen to her mother crying – sobbing in the room next to her. I wasn't consoling her or asking her how she was feeling. All I was thinking about was me – how my life was over and was never to be the same again.

Christmas was coming; the first holiday without my darling Chantal. And oh how she had loved Christmas. We both did and we loved to decorate to the max every year. Christmas music would be playing as we decorated the tree and the house. She also loved to watch Christmas movies. It was a tradition for her. Now, though, it meant nothing to me. I didn't want a tree, I didn't want to decorate, I didn't want to cook a traditional meal…I wanted nothing. December arrived and I needed to get out of the house, so we decided that I would fly home and stay with my parents. Jean and Aleida would fly up a few weeks later to join me and we would have Christmas with our families.

Fuck it was hard. Christmas Eve is always at my parents' and Christmas Day at Jean's parents. We were at my mom and dad's and all my family was there. Everyone but Chantal. I sat, quietly. My mom cooked her traditional meal with all the favorites and Chantal's favorites were Grandma's cabbage rolls and pyroghys. As soon as I cut into that first cabbage roll, I lost it. I ran into one of the bedrooms and sat there and cried. Jean and my brother David came in to console me, but I didn't care what they said because to me, it didn't make a damn bit of difference. My daughter was not there and there was nothing anybody could do about it. Everyone was pretty quiet for the rest of the evening. It was not a typical loud and boisterous family gathering like usual. The next day it was off to the in-laws and it was pretty quiet there as well. I just wanted this Christmas stuff to be over and go back home.

But Christmas wasn't the only thing I had to deal with – her twenty-first birthday was also coming up on the second of January. How the hell was I also going to deal with that? But the load was lightened slightly as some of her girlfriends had decided to get a tattoo in Chantal's honor. Shivon, Colleen, Megan, and Ashlea all had arranged to have a tattoo of the words "I'm Gonna Fly," written in Chantal's handwriting. She had written this in the top column in a poem she wrote to Colleen in high school. The girls were huge Paul Brandt fans and they loved his song, "I'm Gonna Fly." They added a simple design under the words that encompassed Chantal's initials C M D. (You can see a picture in the middle of the book.) The girls invited Aleida and me to also get the tattoo, but I didn't want one because I wasn't ready for something like that yet. But we spent the day in the tattoo shop while they were getting tattooed. My sister Karen and I sat back and watched. We all gathered back at my sister's house afterwards where we laughed and we cried and talked about Chantal.

Soon, seven months had gone by since Chantal's passing and my body was starting to tell me that I had to do something. I had gained weight and every time I got out of bed or up off the couch, my joints would hurt and I could barely move. I started to recognize that it was time to pick myself up and do something. It was spring and flowers were out so I began to go out for walks. After I showered, I would do my hair and put on a little bit of make up and waterproof mascara, but no eyeliner. I was still crying all the time and I didn't want my eyes to get black from it. It was good to move and feel the fresh air, but I was still a walking zombie. My eyes were sad and I didn't smile or laugh. I was a different person.

I started to search for things that could help me. I looked online and at the bookstore for books about how to deal with grief. I really wanted to find something that had been written by a parent who had also lost a child to cancer, but I couldn't find anything. One book had written by a parent who'd lost their child to an accident and this helped a little, but I wanted something that talked about the same kind of loss – loss to cancer. I found a book about the stages of grief called, O*n Grief and Grieving: Finding the Meaning of Grief through the Five Stages of Loss* by Elisabeth Kübler-Ross and David Kessler. This helped give me some understanding of what I was going through. And I also found a few other books that I recommend called: A*nd A Sword Shall Pierce Your Heart: Moving from Despair to Meaning after the Death of a Child* and U*nattended Sorrow* by Stephen Levine. Even though these books provided me with some understanding, I felt it wasn't enough. I needed something more. There were days where I just wanted to end it because I wanted so much to be with Chantal, but I knew I couldn't do that to Jean and Aleida.

Friends and family had repeatedly told me that they did not want me to give up my music – that I needed to get back to it. But I didn't care. I wasn't the same person and my thought was that I would never sing or play again. How could I? Music is supposed to make you feel good and I was not feeling good about anything. I'd lost my daughter and life sucked.

So I thought I needed a retreat of some kind – something where they helped people deal with their grief. I kind of found some things, but nothing truly appealed to me. And for some reason, in my search I came across a music business conference that was going to be taking place in Courtenay, just two hours from where we lived. It was music and I still didn't feel like myself, so I kind of brushed it off. But then I found myself going back to it. Something was telling me that this was what I had to do to start moving forward and putting my life back together again. Finally, I decided that I was going to go and so I registered.

If I had been my regular, bubbly self, I would have been a way more fun person. I'm very outgoing and I love to talk to people. But this time, I was very quiet. I'm sure I came off as shy or an introvert, and when I look back I wish it could have been different. I had my CDs with me and I met and talked with a lot of people – industry and other artists. When asked what I was doing with my music, I simply said, "Nothing right now, 'cause I just lost my daughter and I'm trying to build my life again." Of course people were very sympathetic. And it was one part of the start of my healing process.

But it wasn't enough. I needed something more – something to help me understand why my daughter had to go through what she did and then pass away. One day I was looking through the newspaper and there it was. It was a business card advertisement that had been there week after week, but I'd never seen it before until that day. It was an advertisement for a hypnotherapist – a person who could help you with weight loss, quitting smoking, and dealing with grief. I didn't like counselors or support groups, so this appealed to me. Something told me that this was what I had to do, and I called to set up an appointment.

I met Barbara Adelborg; clinical hypnotherapist, had an hour-session and continued to see her on a regular basis for the next two years. If it weren't for Barb, I don't think I would have returned to being "Shelly." Ever.

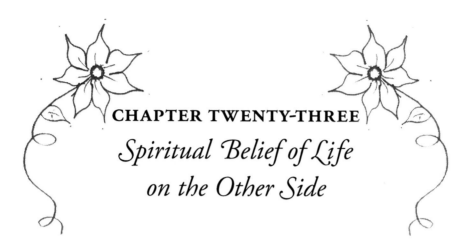

CHAPTER TWENTY-THREE

Spiritual Belief of Life on the Other Side

I FEEL I HAVE TO BACK up here and give some background as to how I came to understand and believe in life on the other side and in the workings of the universe. Not everyone shares the same belief values, which is okay, but I want to share what worked and continues to work for me.

I was born and raised Roman Catholic and I raised my children in the religion as well. All through my school years I always questioned passages from the Bible. I questioned why people went to church. I never felt comfortable with religion. So why did I raise my children Catholic and send them to a Catholic school? It was the thing to do. I did. So my kids went too. I rarely went to church, though. Once in a while I would attend but was always reminded of why I disliked to go so I just stopped going.

About fifteen years ago, while we were still living in Peace River, my friend Cara and her sister Heather were talking about how they had attended some sessions with a medium. A medium? What's that? Over the years I had heard about people you could go to, to talk to people on the "other side," but I never really paid that much attention to it. So I asked, "What is a medium?" A medium is a person who can communicate with or act as a channel for spiritual beings who have passed, to talk to those of us who are still physical beings. Heather was just starting to learn that she was becoming a medium and she was attending these sessions to try to understand how and why these spiritual beings were visiting her. Cara also gave me a book by John Edwards, a very famous medium, to help me understand mediums and life on the other side. Little did I know that this was the beginning of preparing me for what I would experience later in life.

I became intrigued and wanted to learn more, so I attended a session where Heather was doing a group reading. What happens is that you have a group of people in a room with the medium, and then people on the other side start giving her messages that will connect with someone in the room. If you have ever gone to someone for a "reading" and are asked questions, then he or she is not a true medium. A true medium is given "clues" from the person on the other side with which the person on this side can connect. Heather started saying, "I have a man and he is telling me that he is okay – that he is no longer suffering and that you don't have to keep wearing your wedding ring." That connected with a woman in the audience. The medium continued with more information and the more she said, the more it connected with the woman. I know Heather quite well and there was no way she could have been familiar with that information. I became a believer.

And so I continued to educate myself by reading more books about life on the other side and how the universe works. When we made the move to Vancouver Island, I was able to immerse myself in it even more. This was what I needed and this was what I felt was right. I no longer believed in organized religion.

When Chantal was sick, we had tried Reiki treatments and we were introduced to tarot cards. Now some say this is hocus pocus or witchcraft, but once you have an understanding or belief of life on the other side and how the "spirit world" works, it all makes sense. "Spirit world" does not mean demons and ghosts like some like to believe. "Spirit world" or "the other side" is where our souls go once we leave our bodies in the physical world.

I firmly believe that I was introduced to this and kept learning about it to prepare me for Chantal's passing.

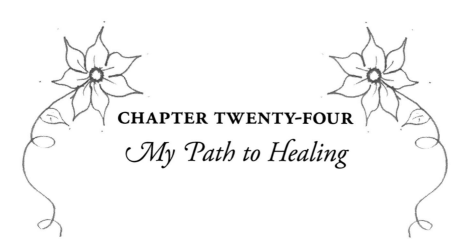

CHAPTER TWENTY-FOUR

My Path to Healing

IN MY HYPNOTHERAPY SESSIONS WITH BARB, we talked about life on the other side and about the universe. I'm sure if I hadn't been on board about all this before, I probably would have said, "Well okay, lady. See you later!"

Even though I had an understanding of life on the other side, I was still angry... angry that my daughter had to leave this physical world at the age of only twenty. That she had to suffer so much through brain cancer. Angry that I could no longer see her, hug her, and hear her infectious laugh. I was heartbroken and I was MAD. Every weekly session with Barb would start with how I was feeling that day, and then we would work on those emotions as Barb took me into a state of hypnosis. It was when I was in this relaxed state that she would ask me why I felt the way I did and then guide me to different visualizations to help me cope with those emotions. Many different techniques were used and quite honestly, because of my state at the time, I can't really remember the exact techniques used. I do remember, though, that in every session I had the freedom to scream, cry, swear – whatever I had to do to get it out.

After a while, my anger started to slowly fade and I became more accepting of Chantal's passing. I was starting to understand and receive signs from her that she was okay. It was the coolest thing sometimes, and it's hard to explain unless you believe and understand it.

As I said earlier, my friends and family were encouraging me to return to music. I had attended the music business conference and in my sessions with Barb, she also encouraged me to return to my music. In our sessions, while I was under hypnosis, she would guide me to walk downstairs, pick up my guitar, and start to play. In the first few sessions, I stopped at the point of picking up my guitar, because I didn't feel I was ready. It still took me a while, but one day, I went downstairs, looked at my guitar, picked it up, and started to play. I then realized how much I missed playing music and how much it was a part of me. I had not played or sung for about a year, so I was pretty rusty. Playing the guitar came back no problem, but my vocal chords had shrunk so I needed to exercise them to get my full voice back. I started searching for a vocal teacher or a vocal program and I found a great vocal program, ordered it, and practiced the exercises every day. Within two weeks, I had a full voice back and it was even better than before, because I had learned some new techniques that improved my vocal abilities.

I had gained a lot of weight and my muscles and joints were sore from sitting around, so I joined a gym and started working with a personal trainer. My first session was the weigh-in and measurements. I did not want to get on that scale. When I did, I saw that I was 175 pounds, and I started to cry. Not only because I was 175 pounds but because that was what I had weighed just before Chantal was born. The significance at that point – I don't know. I attended the gym three days a week and started slowly. Next thing you know I was joining boot camp. I was moving more and then the weight started to come off. It was good.

But...I still missed my daughter. Immensely.

I was getting back into my music, I was exercising, my husband and I were starting to become a couple again, and I was getting re-involved in Aleida's life. But all the while, I still had the heaviness in my heart and the sadness in my eyes. I felt I was just going through the motions of moving forward with my life.

At some point and for some reason, I decided to close Chantal's bedroom door. I would still go in every once in a while, because her room still had her smell. She'd had her favorite hoody, and I would sit on her bed and breathe in her scent. I picked up her brush to touch her hair, which had been left in the bristles. I looked through her albums of pictures. I had left the room untouched. Nothing had been moved.

I told Barb how I had closed the door, so we worked through how I could eventually open it up again. She guided me, while under hypnosis, to walk up the stairs and go to Chantal's bedroom door. She asked how I was feeling at that moment and to explain why I had that feeling. Then she would assist me to look at it from a different perspective and provided further guidance to make peace with opening the bedroom door.

I actually hated living in our house at that time, because the reminders were there – every day in every room. I didn't even want to sit on the living room furniture because she had laid there in agony when the chemo treatments had caused that excruciating leg pain. I couldn't even go into the main floor bathroom or the bathroom by the bedrooms, because I couldn't stand the flashbacks of the many times I had to rush her into the washroom to try to get her on the toilet because of the urgency to pee. Or the times she'd sat in her wheelchair brushing her hair and clumps of hair had fallen out. Jean or Aleida would clean those bathrooms. Thank goodness we had an ensuite in our bedroom. In my sessions with Barb, we talked about this and she took me through steps of how to deal with it. Slowly, I made my way into the bathrooms and we painted the living room a different color and moved things around a bit.

I continued on my spiritual healing journey by reading more books by famous author Doreen Virtue about life on the other side. I needed to understand more – I needed more information. With the combination of the hypnotherapy sessions and the reading I was doing I was starting to become a little more accepting of Chantal's passing.

A year had passed and I still had not returned to work. I felt I couldn't focus and I was trying to figure out what the hell I was going to do with my life. And I couldn't sleep. I was up all hours of the night because I couldn't close my eyes. As soon as I closed them, the flashbacks started and I couldn't handle it. So I would watch TV until four or five o'clock in the morning until my eyes could no longer stay open and then sleep until noon. Some people return to work within a few months because they feel they have to keep themselves busy, but I couldn't do that. I wanted to deal with my grief, and besides I was also trying to build myself back up physically as well. My body was exhausted from all the stress and I felt that I had to get myself healthy before adding back the stress of work.

October 17, 2009 – first anniversary of her passing. I couldn't believe that it had been a year. A year! Another big event that I had to deal with, but Barb once again assisted me through it. Chantal's friends back home were honoring her by going out and enjoying two of her favorite things – Caesars and pizza. I thought that was a wonderful thing, so now every year on the anniversary of her passing and on her birthday we have Caesars and pizza. They say that all the "firsts" are the hardest and they are. We had already experienced the first Christmas and first birthday and now it was the first year.

I continued with my sessions with Barb, played music more, started to go out again, and continued with my exercising. Sleep was still eluding me, but it was starting to get better. I still watched TV until I fell asleep, but instead of it being four or five in the morning it would be two or three.

My healing was continuing to be a lot of work and I still went into Chantal's room to cry and breathe in her scent. That was the biggest part of why I left things untouched. I was afraid that if I packed up anything or cleaned anything that I would lose her scent. It was the last physical thing I had of her and I was not about to let that go. Her room remained untouched for the next three years.

In July of 2010, my long-term disability benefit was getting cut off and I made the decision not to return to my job. I just felt I couldn't return to a nine-to-five office job environment. I wasn't the same person I had been and dealing with people – sometimes difficult people (the clients), was not something I could do. In that job you needed to have a backbone and I didn't have one. I was still a blubbering, sad mother who had lost a child. Music was actually healing for me and the environment that music provided me was one of support, love, and encouragement. That's what I needed.

Barb, my hypnotherapist, continued to be my savior. Jean and Aleida could see my progress so they decided to go see her as well.

They didn't have as many sessions as I did, but they were grateful for the ones they did have as these helped them as well. All three of us were on a spiritual healing journey. The more I learned the more I shared, to get them involved as well. All three of us were experiencing a deeper understanding of life on the other side, and we were learning to pay attention and recognize signs from Chantal's spirit that she was close by. That was the hardest thing to accept – that her physical presence was gone, but her spiritual presence was still with us.

January 2, 2011, Chantal would have been twenty-three and I felt I needed to give her a birthday present. I had a song that was swirling around in my head and I knew that if I wrote it, it would be a great birthday gift to her. I went down in the basement in my music area and didn't come out until the song was completed. Late that night, I had my song, "I Know You're Here." I have not officially recorded it, but I do have a YouTube video of me singing it. You can visit my YouTube channel: http://www.youtube.com/ShellyDubois1 to listen to it.

I remember our very first reading. It was with Heather (the medium I spoke about earlier), and it was over the phone. Spirit has no specified locations or boundaries.

So we put Heather on speaker-phone and put the receiver on the kitchen table. She said a prayer and then warned us that Chantal might not come through at first, and Chantal didn't. But Jean's grandpa did and it really caught him off guard. Heather said an old gentleman was coming through. She described him as a bigger man with pure white hair, and she said that he was showing her a watch. (Jean's grandpa had repaired watches and clocks.) But it was all okay. Eventually Chantal made her way through and her message to us was that she was fine. She said that she was keeping her hair short because she liked it that way and that it was very peaceful where she was. Jean and I cried. It was hard to hear this but at the same time comfort-ing. She was not dead and gone and never to be heard from again. Her spirit was still alive and she was communicating with us from the other side. We still had a connection, and that was the part that was comforting to me and to Jean.

I had also met Erin – a medium and tarot card reader who was helping with my healing as well. Periodically I would visit Erin for a reading as would Jean and Aleida. Not only did we receive messages from our spiritual guides, but each time Chantal would also come through and give us a message.

Chantal had loved dolphins – I don't know why. She just did. I had come to a point in my music where I had put a band together, and I was about to set out on a two- week tour so I had a reading with Erin before I left. Chantal came through and said that whenever I saw dolphins or a feather that would mean that she was around.

As my band and I drove into Alberta and we were on the divided highway between Jasper and Edmonton, there was a trailer-truck sitting on the opposite side of the road. And it had a picture of two large dolphins on it. Before each performance, when I got out of the van, there was a feather on the ground. She was there – helping me continue with my dream of performing music. I actually started to feel her presence.

I remember a particular session with Barb in which Chantal came through and Barb said, "She's talking about a song that is popular on the radio right now that she likes. Something about beer and crazy people." And yes there was a song called "People Are Crazy," but a line in the chorus went: "God is great, beer is good, and people are crazy."

After I left the session, I got in my car, started it up, and that song was playing on the radio. Billy Currington's song "People Are Crazy" was not released to radio until March 2n^{d}, 2009, AFTER Chantal had passed away. But the album it was on, *Little Bit of Everything*, was released on October 14, 2008, while Chantal was in the hospital.

So it was incidents like this and many others that were continual confirmation to me that there is life on the other side. Chantal wasn't with me physically any more but she continued to be with me spiritually and does so to this day.

Life continued on and I was becoming more involved in my music, while Jean continued his job at the local hospital. Aleida completed school and graduated with a whack of scholarships to go to university for Jazz Studies. I was trying to make some money with my music, but as anybody in the music business knows, it just costs you money. We were still only on one income, money was getting very tight, and we had to do something. Jean took a job in Fort McMurray, and in the spring of 2012 we moved. I was now forced to pack up Chantal's room.

How was I going to do this? H*er scent! I'm going to lose her scent!* But the last clothes that she had worn and her favorite hoody, which I had kept smelling for the past four years, I packed into the cedar chest that her pépère had made for her. I packed as much as I could in there and those poor movers had to lug it down the stairs and out to the truck. I cried so hard going through her clothes. I just couldn't decide what to get rid of. I didn't want to get rid of anything, but I knew I had to. Aleida kept some clothing and I also kept a few items, but the rest had to go. So I quickly threw them into a garbage bag and shipped them off to Salvation Army. I kept all her jewelry because I wanted to eventually be able to wear some myself or give some away to her friends. I still have this chest of clothes, jewelry, pictures, and other odds and ends.

The house we rented in Fort McMurray was very small and we only had the top floor. The garage was our storage room, so now all of Chantal's belongings were in a cedar chest out in the garage. I kept it accessible.

We only stayed a year in Fort McMurray and then we moved closer to Edmonton to Fort Saskatchewan where we are settled today.

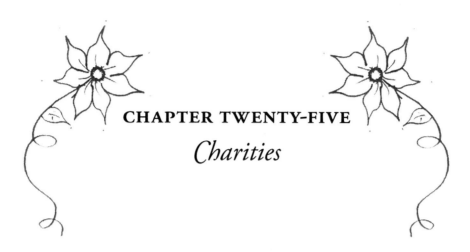

CHAPTER TWENTY-FIVE

Charities

BECAUSE OF THE GENEROSITY, LOVE, AND support that were shown to us when we were going through Chantal's cancer battle, while we were living in British Columbia I worked with an organization called BCCCPA – British Columbia Child Cancer Parents' Association. BCCCPA operates out of Vancouver and gives financial help to families with a child who is battling cancer. The founder and executive director of the association is an incredible human being who has lost *two* children to cancer and continues to work with families facing that battle today.

Since moving back to Alberta, I've been working with the Helping Families Handle Cancer Foundation out of Calgary. It also offers financial help to families with a child battling cancer. The executive director is a childhood cancer survivor and has dedicated her time to easing financial stress for these families. As of August 2015 I became a board member of Helping Families Helping Cancer.

I perform shows in dedication to these charities and have raised approximately $20,000 as well as awareness of what happens when a child is diagnosed with cancer. It is my goal to travel across Canada performing shows and raising hundreds of thousands of dollars to help provide financial support to families with a cancer-stricken child.

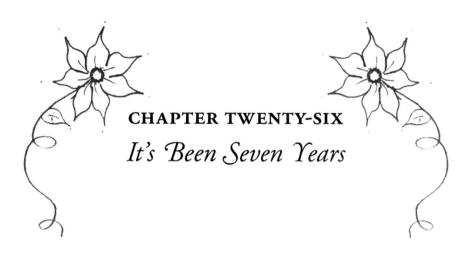

CHAPTER TWENTY-SIX

It's Been Seven Years

ALONG WITH OTHER CHERISHED ITEMS, CHANTAL'S ashes are still in an urn in a corner cabinet that we purchased especially for the purpose. Beside the cabinet is a table with her picture and the candle that was at her funeral service. The candle is lit every year on the anniversary of her passing. Some articles of clothing, her jewelry, pictures, and other things we hold dear are in the cedar chest, which I still go into every once in a while. Every birthday and every anniversary of her passing, we still have Caesars and pizza.

I started to write this book a year ago, but as I got closer to writing about when her health really started to decline I had to stop. I was not prepared to relive those moments in my life, and I was afraid that if I did I would set myself back. Things were progressing well for me and I wanted to keep it that way. I knew there would be a right time – that I would come to a place in my life where I would have the strength to finish writing the book. I have continued to do more spiritual work, and now I feel that I am in total touch with the universe and with how the spirit world works.

I worked with Barb again to help me come to a place where I could write. Eventually, in one session she said, "You have to write about Chantal's legacy." And that was it. That was the moment I realized

– yes, I have to write about Chantal. To tell the story of how brave she was and that she was a fighter.

I have come to fully accept that Chantal had a purpose here, as we all do and that she had to leave early as her time in the physical world was done. I still experience her presence every once in a while, and I receive signs that she's with me.

My heart still aches but not as much, and I still have my moments where I really miss her and have a good cry. Sometimes I can talk about her with a huge smile on my face and other times it's with sadness and tears, but that's okay. Grief has no end, and it shouldn't. I've lost a child – a human being to whom I gave birth, and who I nurtured and loved. And we shared a very special bond.

I'm back to being "Shelly" again, something I never thought I would be.

I will always cherish the time Chantal and I had together in this physical life and I look forward to the day that I will join her on the other side where we will be reunited.

I have one last message from Chantal, which I received in my readings that I would like to share with you. She said:

It's not *impossible*
it's
I'M POSSIBLE

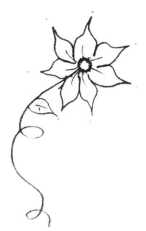
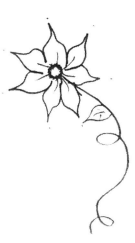

REFERENCES

Avastin (bevacizumab)

A drug used alone or with other drugs to treat certain types of cervical, colorectal, lung, kidney, ovarian, fallopian tube, and primary peritoneal cancer, and glioblastoma (a type of brain cancer). It is also being studied in the treatment of other types of cancer. Bevacizumab binds to a protein called vascular endothelial growth factor (VEGF). This may prevent the growth of new blood vessels that tumors need to grow. It is a type of antiangiogenesis agent and a type of monoclonal antibody.

Source: http://www.cancer.gov/publications/dictionaries/cancer-terms?cdrid=46115

Dexamethasone

A synthetic adrenal corticosteroid with potent anti-inflammatory properties. In addition to binding to specific nuclear steroid receptors, dexamethasone also interferes with NF-kB activation and apoptotic pathways. This agent lacks the salt-retaining properties of other related adrenal hormones.

Source: http://www.cancer.gov/publications/dictionaries/cancer-drug?CdrID=39789

Irinotecan Hydrocloride (Campto)

The hydrochloride salt of a semisynthetic derivative of camptothecin, a cyto-toxic, quinoline-based alkaloid extracted from the Asian tree Camptotheca acuminata. Irinotecan, a prodrug, is converted to a biologically active metabolite 7-ethyl-10-hydroxy-camptothecin (SN-38) by a carboxylesterase-converting enzyme. One thousand-fold more potent than its parent compound irinotecan, SN-38 inhibits topoisomerase I activity by stabilizing the cleavable complex between topoisomerase I and DNA, resulting in DNA breaks that inhibit DNA replication and trigger apoptotic cell death. Because ongoing DNA synthesis is necessary for irinotecan to exert its cytotoxic effects, it is classified as an S-phase-specific agent.

Neulasta (pegfilgrastim)
This is a drug used to decrease the risk of infections in certain patients undergoing chemotherapy by stimulating bone marrow to produce white blood cells.

Temodal (temozolomide)
A triazene analog of dacarbazine with antineoplastic activity. As a cytotoxic alkylating agent, temozolomide is converted at physiologic pH to the short-lived active compound, monomethyl triazeno imidazole carboxamide (MTIC). The cytotoxicity of MTIC is due primarily to methylation of DNA at the O6 and N7 positions of guanine, resulting in inhibition of DNA replication. Unlike dacarbazine, which is metabolized to MITC only in the liver, temozolomide is metabolized to MITC at all sites. Temozolomide is administered orally and penetrates well into the central nervous system.
Source: http://www.cancer.gov/publications/dictionaries/cancer-drug?CdrID=41671

Glioblastoma Multiforme
A fast-growing type of central nervous system tumor that forms from glial (supportive) tissue of the brain and spinal cord and has cells that look very different from normal cells. Glioblastoma multiforme usually occurs in adults and affects the brain more often than the spinal cord. Also called GBM, glioblastoma, and grade IV astrocytoma.
Source: http://www.cancer.gov/publications/dictionaries/cancer-terms?cdrid=45699

Radiation Therapy
Radiation therapy uses high-energy radiation to shrink tumors and kill cancer cells. X-rays, gamma rays, and charged particles are types of radiation used for cancer treatment. The radiation may be delivered by a machine outside the body (external-beam radiation therapy), or it may come from

radioactive material placed in the body near cancer cells (internal radiation therapy, also called brachytherapy).Systemic radiation therapy uses radioactive substances, such as radioactive iodine, that travel in the blood to kill cancer cells. About half of all cancer patients receive some type of radiation therapy sometime during the course of their treatment.

Radiation therapy kills cancer cells by damaging their DNA (the molecules inside cells that carry genetic information and pass it from one generation to the next). Radiation therapy can either damage DNA directly or create charged particles (free radicals) within the cells that can in turn damage the DNA.

Cancer cells whose DNA is damaged beyond repair stop dividing or die. When the damaged cells die, they are broken down and eliminated by the body's natural processes.

Radiation therapy can also damage normal cells, leading to side effects.

Doctors take potential damage to normal cells into account when planning a course of radiation therapy. The amount of radiation that normal tissue can safely receive is known for all parts of the body. Doctors use this information to help them decide where to aim radiation during treatment.

Radiation therapy is sometimes given with curative intent (that is, with the hope that the treatment will cure a cancer, either by eliminating a tumor, preventing cancer recurrence, or both). In such cases, radiation therapy may be used alone or in combination with surgery, chemotherapy, or both.

Source: http://www.cancer.gov/about-cancer/treatment/
types/radiation-therapy/radiation-fact-sheet

ABOUT THE AUTHOR

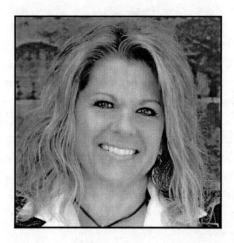

SHELLY DUBOIS (NÉE DUPERRON) WAS BORN in Peace River, Alberta, as one of five siblings. At ten years old she began playing music and has been performing in bands since she was thirteen. As a country artist, she enjoys a professional career and has released her music to country music radio in Canada, the United States, and some European countries. A member of the Association of Country Music in Alberta, she was nominated for Female Artist of the Year and Fan's Choice in 2012 and again for Female Artist in 2013. After the passing of her daughter, Shelly joined organizations that offer financial aid to families battling cancer. With her performances she has helped raise awareness and funds for the BC Childhood Cancer Parents Association (BCCCPA) as well as Alberta's Helping Families Handle Cancer Foundation, for which she is a board member. Shelly and her husband Jean have been married for twenty-five years. You can visit her musician website at www.shelly-dubois.com.

CPSIA information can be obtained at www.ICGtesting.com
Printed in the USA
LVOW10s0742120416

483148LV00017B/188/P